Johann Kellerer

Perfume

THE HIDDEN BANE OF YOUR HEALTH

The Insidious Billion-Dollar Business
of Beauty, Sex and Chemicals
that Costs YOUR Health and Money

ISBN-13: 978-1-0814-0341-6
ISBN-10: 1-0814-0341-1

Independently published
Typeset by Amnet systems.

The second edition is a revised version with a few corrections of the original text. And it contains two additional chapters on current topics.

The programs in this book have been included for their instructional value. They have been tested with care but are not guaranteed for any particular purpose and are not intended as medical advice. The publisher does not offer any warranties or representation, nor does it accept any liabilities concerning the programs.

Dedication

*This book is dedicated to the people of all nations, races,
colors, and religions, because on my travels through Western
and Eastern Europe, North and South Africa, Arabia, China
and Southeast Asia, and North and South America I have
repeatedly found that everyone wants the same thing: survival, happiness and the best possible health.*

*This book is about the latter. May it fill a knowledge gap and
thereby make the best possible **possible**.*

Note: This book was translated from German and accordingly,
most references pertain to that country. But the author, having
traveled to many countries and observed similar conditions
everywhere, knows that this situation is a global problem. So,
most of the German references do also apply for other areas,
and even those that do not, are good examples of the most
extensive ongoing home-environment pollution ever.

Table of Contents

Foreword
(if not to say WARNING!)

Dear Reader,

You might not like this book.

You may think that I exaggerate, or that I seem to have been writing this in an emotional state of wrath and revenge. It might appear to be too radical.

Especially if you are a woman who loves perfume, you might even start to hate me. On the other hand, I believe I will express the heartfelt sentiments of the mothers among you.

Men? I guess some of you if you haven't yet been convinced to wear perfume in the form of cologne, aftershave, deodorants, gels, oils, and soaps might absorb the content objectively.

Of course, if you are a chemist, you will most likely try to disprove it by whatever means you can. Chemical companies, perfume producers, and their advertising icons? They will hate me and try to ban this book with complaints and threats.

So, should I only sell this book to mothers, non- chemists, and the few who don't wear perfume?

No way! On the contrary! I want every woman and man in the world to read this book.

I may be seeing my face on 'Wanted' posters soon, though!

So why am I taking this risk?

1. **Without food, we can survive one to three months.**
2. **Without water, five to seven days.**
3. **Without air? A minute or two!**

These three aspects should make it clear that AIR is the most important element that our bodies need to survive.

And what every environmental activist and organic food-fan have long realized, is: the more our food and water is contaminated, the more our health is endangered. The same is true for the quality of the very air that we breathe.

And what 99.9% of the public either does not know or blatantly ignore: chemically produced perfume is a dangerous air pollutant. And it is right here in our homes, offices, and in all parts of our life 24/7 – but often hidden.

These were the arguments that led me years ago to gather and publish the *facts* about perfume. The issue of smoking took countless years before the tobacco industry was put in its place. I think it is now time to clean up the decades of misinformation, viciously indoctrinated into us by the advertising psychologists of the perfume industry, through which we daily poison ourselves and our family, friends, and acquaintances in small, repeated doses out of ignorance.

Johann Kellerer

Knowledge is Power.

FRANCIS BACON
English philosopher (1561–1626)

CHAPTER 1

Perfume, the Legalized Killing Weapon

THE TITLE OF this book is Perfume, the Hidden Bane of your Health. And its provocative subtitle, The Insidious Billion-Dollar Business of Beauty, Sex and Chemicals that Costs Your Health and Money, should leave you in no doubt that I won't mince my words when telling you all there is to be said about perfume – although the multibillion-dollar industry will surely try to dispute the facts I am going to lay in front of you in the following pages.

First and foremost, you need to understand that there is more to know about perfume and about the unfathomable side effects that perfume can have.

So, what can the reader expect from this book? I want to start by going back in time. Looking at the history of perfume, one finds that, at a significant point in history, the fragrance trade took an unexpected turn and developed into a monstrosity that no one could have foreseen. These facts will be presented to you in the next chapter.

Few people are aware of which areas and places and in which products and objects we encounter perfume daily. Continue reading to be blown away.

Theoretically, at one time, if one were to avoid countries that are known for a certain kind of 'perfumey' culture, it wasn't too hard to also avoid contact with perfumes. Unfortunately, this isn't possible anymore. Unless one decides to live in complete solitude somewhere in Tibet, there is no escaping these toxins. 'No man is an island,' as first John Donne and then Ernest Hemingway so accurately stated.

I discovered the truth of this on a recent business trip to Chechnya, a republic which belongs to Russia. According to various sources, Chechnya is an area surrounded by high mountains, with clean air, far away from so-called civilization. We decided to rest in a mountain village, remote and secluded. It seemed the villagers only knew what computers and smartphones were because someone had told them about these mysterious machines. Would you believe what I found when visiting the gents – apart from the evidence of visitors before me? A *wall* of perfume!

No matter how isolated or far away in the backwoods one is located, perfume molecules are everywhere. Even if not transmitted directly to you from your perfume, the minute particles of scent that travel through the atmosphere and infiltrate every niche will surely find their way to you. I will prove this with specific facts.

What else can you expect from this book?

If we are to believe some perfume ads, we are promised a world full of luxury, beauty, and sex, as long as we smell the way we're told to.

"Perfume is like a new dress. It makes you quite simply marvelous," according to a slogan used by the American cosmetics company Estée Lauder to promote its products. Even Coco Chanel tells us: "A woman who doesn't wear perfume has no future."

Perfume, extravagance, luxury, sex, and beauty go hand in hand – this is what the ads make us believe every day. Much can be said about that: they are things that are usually only told off the record. More importantly, very few know about the long-term side effects of perfume. A delicate perfume, the epitome of culture, can lead to severe allergies, and what's more, it is the real reason for many illnesses from which many people suffer, perhaps even you, without knowing their real cause.

Reactions to perfume creep insidiously into our system and take hold in a malicious and underhand manner. After all, the fragrance tricks us into thinking that our appearance can be defined by how we smell.

Alas! This false friend, over time, turns out to be an appalling fiend. There is, in reality, a whole conglomeration of illnesses and grievances that are immediately associated with the effects of perfume – there have even been reported deaths from poisoning by perfume.

Because of the almost unbelievable nature of the information, I am about to reveal, I have to ask my readers to buckle up. This is going to be a wild rollercoaster ride. It is fair to say that you will encounter some surprising truths and maybe even some shocking facts. But it is precisely these facts that will be your weapon. This knowledge can help you sharpen your senses, help you regain them. It will build a stronger foundation for your immune system and create overall a healthier state of being.

The information in this book could even be responsible for completely changing your life for the better. Dramatic as it may sound, knowing the truth about perfume can be a matter of life and death, which is why I decided to write this book. How can we stand by and watch greedy directors fill their pockets and collect large profits while knowingly condoning the premature deaths of millions of people?

This book, therefore, was written out of concern. In my opinion, it isn't fair to keep you, the reader, out of the loop. We all have a right to know the truth. Indeed, your well-being depends on it! Many grievances which we take as a given – tiredness, illness, lethargy – shouldn't be a given. Sure enough, with just a few small steps and the right decisions, these can be eliminated.

To this end, I am offering you solutions in the last chapters of this book to problems that may be affecting you.

As a side note – I believe that "bad news" should only be broadcast if and when a simple, immediate and applicable solution can be presented simultaneously. You will find exactly those kinds of solutions later in this book.

There have already been some remarkable movements against this perfume mania. Even some legislative bodies have become aware of it. More importantly, you can take some small actions to make a big difference. The motto here is:

Something can be done about it.

The crucial question is: *what* can we and *what* can you specifically and actively do about it? This is the question I will answer thoroughly later in this text.

So, to whom are the following pages addressed? They are directed to anyone who comes into contact with perfume. In today's world, that is basically everyone. In particular, I would like to address this book to mothers who don't get enough praise. Mothers always have and will always make continuous efforts to ensure the well-being of their children. Nobody gives more to the family than a mother. The applause for mothers should be long and hard. Perhaps that is why they are the most important readers for me – every one of them should read this book.

But let me rephrase that. Anyone concerned about his or her own wellbeing – and the wellbeing of those they love and to whom they wish well – should read this book. Once you know the truth and have the facts, you can immediately go about changing your life and effectively helping your environment. The motto here is:

Knowledge is power!

Once you know which substances cause what problems, you can become active right away.

A last word before we start on our ride: It is important to me that a book, even a non-fiction book, should be easily understood and shouldn't contain technical terms which probably only one percent of the readers would understand. Complex chemical formulas and technical terms have been added only as side notes. This way I am catering for experts as well as for ordinary people, who can if they choose, ignore these notes.

So far, so good: now, let's get the facts on the table. As a first question, let us ask ourselves: Who invented the first perfume? Whom do we thank for this concoction?

Usually, when one homes in on the originator, one discovers more than just one secret. Let's get to it.

*History: a collection of facts
which could have been avoided.*

STANISLAW JERZY LEC
Polish poet and aphorist (1909–1966)

Chapter 2

A Short History of Perfume

IF YOU WANT to sift through a subject to illuminate it, nothing is as enlightening as a look at its history. Provided one has accurate sources, history reveals a lot and clarifies for us the puppet-masters behind the scenes and the causes of a specific outcome, as well as the exact time and place of its creation. Often, history even tells us about the original intentions of those masterminds behind the scenes, and so we would always do well to consult history before we make any judgments on a subject. Let us treat ourselves to this luxury, and at least begin to examine the history of perfume.

We encounter three men behind the scenes, three types of masterminds, quite early on, which will not leave us astonished.

In this chapter, we can look forward to some surprises, too.

What exactly is a perfume?

The word "perfume" (in German "Parfüm," French "perfume," English "perfume" or "fragrance") derives from the

Latin term *fumum*, which means the same as "fumes" or "smoke."

As early as the days of the ancient Romans, burnt incense was used to create pleasant odors and to delight the nose and tickle it with something special. The desire to provide our nose with fragrances is ancient; we can trace the path much further back. There were perfumes already among the ancient Indians, among the ancient Greeks – and the Egyptians.

The Secrets of the Egyptian Priests

Perfume was already in fashion back in the time of the ancient Egyptians. The pharaoh Hatshepsut (1476–1448 BC) believed in the use of fragrances. "Hatshepsut" means "the first of the most distinguished women" – but wait: a *woman* on the king's throne?

This was indeed an extraordinary phenomenon. Since only men could sit on the Egyptian throne, Hatshepsut would often dress up as a man. There is no doubt that she even attached a beard at public ceremonies to be accepted as ruler.

From where in ancient Egyptian culture, did perfume originate? How did the knowledge of perfume get into the Pharaoh's hands?

To answer this question, we must go directly into the mysterious passages of the pyramids and the hidden tombs on the banks of the Nile. In them may be found the most magnificent graves of the greatest kings of history, which still impress us today. They were usually only accessible through twisted passages, which were sometimes spiked with booby traps. They contained shafts and false chambers so that a robber risked nothing less than his life if he wanted to steal the treasures of the royal tombs. The greatest secrets were hidden in burial chambers, which were only accessible to the priests. Not only were they filled with glittering gold and immeasurably precious treasures, but more importantly, arcane spells were incised on the coffins. Such engraved incantations allowed the dead to avoid certain traps in the hereafter, after their resurrection.

The ancient Egyptians believed in life after death. They assumed that the soul, called *Ba* or *Ka*, would be resurrected together with the body. Therefore, it was essential to prepare the body so that it did not fall to pieces and could be re-used. It was precisely for this purpose that specific chemical knowledge was needed.

Egyptian priests, who served the god of the dead, opened a corpse and removed the organs. Even the brain was removed: if we are to believe some ancient writings, it was extracted through the nose with oblong tweezers. The organs were placed into clay jars, and carefully sealed, but only after they had been treated. The empty body-shell itself was now filled with a solution of sodium, for which the exact chemical formula to this day remains uncertain. This process was accompanied by intense and pungent smells, repetitive sing-song spells, and the murmurs of the priests. All the priests wore fearsome masks, most likely to serve as some form of protection against the terrible smells. At any rate, aromatic neutralizers against the stench and odors in the death chambers were already used in these early days.

The neutralizer? The solution? Good odors! Perfumes!

And so, a few thousand years ago, in ancient Egypt, we encounter complex mixtures of incense, myrrh, and rose petals mixed with oils, wine, and other ingredients. So, it was death that brought us the first perfumes, perfumes intended to enhance lives in the years to come.

The mummifying priests probably added them to the body parts and rubbed the corpses with them. A priest worked for hours on a corpse that had most likely already started to rot. Not all the waters of the Nile, nor other waters of the world, could remove the stench from the priest's garments and hands. One can assume that the priests themselves made use of the perfumes to remove or mask the odor that clung to them. Despite this, priority was always given to the dead. The bodies of the kings and their wives had to be preserved under all circumstances. They were carefully anointed so that they could arrive as perfectly as possible in the hereafter.

The ancient Egyptians distinguished between a kind of hell, with steaming fire lakes and poisonous pools, and an area which today we might call heaven. In any case, the priests taught that after death, one had possibilities of transformation: one could become a bird or a star or take hold of a new animal or human body.[1]

However, the priests kept this knowledge well-hidden and only shared it if one had passed a test, and one's deeds were found to be "good."

They still believed that the body that was left behind was of utmost importance. Therefore, secret spells were carefully carved or painted on the coffin walls and the walls of the tombs so that the (old) body wouldn't decay. This, of course, was achieved with the help of chemistry and fragrances.

The knowledge of how to neutralize odors and bring about good smells came into the hands of the ancient Egyptian aristocracy and the royal court. We do not have an accurate account of how the know-how was passed on, or by whom. One could imagine, though, that, with the prospect of making money, the priests would happily sell this knowledge to noble, aristocratic women who were seeking the attention of the men. It had already been discovered in ancient Egypt that certain fragrances could exert a unique effect on some men. So, we know that during Hatshepsut's reign – and presumably earlier, though this can't be proven – perfumes came into fashion. One could assume that there was a market for this, as the ingredients of some perfumes had to be procured from the most distant parts of what was then the known world.

Whole caravans moved in the four heavenly directions and acquired the necessary ingredients for the ancient perfumes. An unimaginably extended trade existed even then, with smart merchants and courageous adventurers buying the components in foreign countries and selling them to make a profit. Their customers were Pharaoh Hatshepsut, amongst other noble ladies.

An old Egyptian papyrus, a sort of letter, addressed to Hatshepsut, reads:

> *"Heaven and earth shall overflow with incense, and the scent shall be in the house of princes. Pure and immaculate the ointment for the divine limbs should be."*[2]

What is meant by "ointment for divine limbs"? It is a reference to the scented lotions that were meant for Hatshepsut herself.

We, therefore, see that thousands of years ago, a regular beauty industry already existed. As is the case today, recipes and formulas were jealously guarded and treated as "secret knowledge." Every possible flower, plant, tree, and animal was examined as to whether it could be used in perfumes. The most known was the famous Kyphi, a fragrance made from a mixture of incense, myrrh, resin, sandalwood, rose petals, fatty oils, wine, and other ingredients. Kyphi (an exact translation is unknown) was produced in the laboratory-workshops within the temples and initially served in sacrificial worship while the priests recited words from their holy scriptures. It was later when Kyphi was adopted by the Arabs, Greeks, and Romans that it was also used in wine, or to rub directly onto the skin.

The number of ingredients expanded steadily from ten to fifty, using incense, myrrh, cedar, ginger, various herbs, raisins, the bark of cinnamon trees, juniper berries, parts of the cypress tree, honey and many more. Each mixture had its secret recipe.

So, while it started as a scent used for dead people, it was the living people who adorned themselves with the scents and fragrances of embalming perfume for years to come. Even the gorgeous Nefertiti is known to have used perfumes. Nefertiti, whose name means "the beautiful one has come," was the wife of the chief Pharaoh Akhenaten, who ruled in the fourteenth century BC. The Great Royal Wife (one of Nefertiti's titles) was known to have used perfumes to increase her appeal. Her efforts were rewarded. Nefertiti played a significant role in the religious and political circles of ancient Egypt. Among other things, she strengthened the position of women and was made co-regent by the Pharaoh.

Indian Fragrances

To research and write a small thesis about the role of perfumes in all past cultures would be an exciting task, but that is not my intention. We should at least look to India, though, as here too the priests played a decisive role. Incense was already used by the Brahmins, the Indian priestly caste. Incense, fragrances, and, in all likelihood, drug-like substances were used by priests of different cultures to put the mind into an unconscious state to create a lasting impression. Believers were "transported" into a different place by the fumes of the fragrances, giving them the feeling of having left the here and now.

Perhaps too little attention has been drawn to the fact that priests can also be villains. Many Brahmins asked for a fee, and this hocus-pocus was costly. The gods had to be bribed, and incense played a crucial role in sacrificial rituals. In ancient Indian medicine, incense was called Salai Guggal and had been in use for over 5,000 years before our time, which tells us that it originated in India. Salai Guggal or frankincense as we call it today traveled along the ancient incense road via Yemen and Syria, over top-secret and vigilantly monitored trading routes to all regions of the world. It could then be exchanged for gold and money.

The Brahmins used this incense, as well as many other secretly kept fragrances, which were sometimes laced with all sorts of drug-like substances. The believer who inhaled these substances was left thoroughly impressed – and so was willing to pay an excessive amount of money. Many Brahmins quickly forgot their doctrine of the transience of matter when it came to fill their pockets.

Nothing compares to the lavishness that was displayed around the Brahmins. The most unlikely superstitions were encouraged – the priests could make infertile women fertile again, forgive sins, predict the future, and speak with the gods. They were masters of prestidigitation, and, with the use of fragrances, they had the people hooked.

"Men were put into service to simulate madness and to confess that their fate was the punishment for their avarice against the priests," the historian Will Durant tells us.

Every disease, every dream, every legal matter, was exploited by the priests and turned into money. Incense was regularly used to impress the faithful. But we now know that all these "incense plants" were, to a certain extent, the harbinger of perfumes.

The Brahmins were untouchable due to their unique bond with the gods, and only they could interpret the will of the gods correctly. Some Brahmins even enjoyed sexual privileges over all the brides of their territory. The first night belonged to them. Other women were given the impression that if they spent one night in a holy Brahmin temple, they could be cured of their infertility. Whoever killed a Brahmin had to die. If someone killed a warrior, however, one had to pay a Brahmin a thousand cows for atonement. Nowhere did greed flourish as much as in this Indian "priest" caste. Religious beliefs were stifled under this power- and sex-driven elite.

We have further heard of perfume in combination with the famous Kama Sutra. *Kama Sutra* means "verses of desire." It is a handbook of eroticism, love, and sex. The work was written about 200-300 AD, though nothing is known about the life of the author. All kinds of sexual positions are openly described in this work, in shocking detail. Readers are enlightened about virgins, wives, the wives of other men, and courtesans, ironically in a rather chaste manner.

The author explains the art of embracing and the variations of kissing. He sets rules for biting with teeth and describes the habits of men during sexual intercourse. The Kama Sutra is an interesting adviser. The writer advises men on the best ways of courting young women and women on the right attitude toward their husbands, distinguishing between young and old wives, the widow that remarries and the one living in a harem. The book further warns about high-class whores and promiscuous women. In short, the book describes the method of finding the right sexual partner and what is required to be a "good lover."

Even the role of perfume and odors is broached, advising men to steer clear of unhealthy and filthy women:

"... every intelligent human being should make use of aromatic substances. Apply scented creams on your body, dab your lips with perfumed wax, polish your teeth thoroughly, put flowers in your hair, and attach them to your clothes."[3]

This leads to the conclusion that perfumes made with natural ingredients had already been in use in ancient India. A link between eroticism, sex, and perfumes existed even then, thousands of years ago.

A 180° turn on the subject took place in our Northern latitudes when a particular genus of man took up the issue of perfume. That brings us to the next episode.

Pharmacists and Alchemists

Perfumes came into our latitudes through the Crusades, a time when some fanatical popes and preachers decided that "unbelievers," "Muslims" and "Islamic dogs" should be banned from Jerusalem in the mid and late Middle Ages (eleventh to fifteenth centuries). Pope Urban II was one of the key individuals during the Crusades. Full of hatred and religious fervor, he preached:

> *"The cradle of our salvation, the fatherland of the Lord, the motherland of religion, has a godless nation in its power. The godless people of the Saracens for a long time have afflicted with their tyranny the holy places where the Lord's feet walked and kept the faithful in slavery and submission. The dogs have entered the sanctuary, and the holiest of holies has been desecrated. The people who reverence the true God are humbled ..."*[4]

As a result, Christian knights and peasants, women and children were inspired to act to return Jerusalem into the bosom of the church. Involuntarily, they came in contact with the partly superior culture of the Orient, where the hygienic standards were much higher and rare fragrances, and spices drifted through the air, unlike in Germany, where one only knew of lavender water.

Lavender water is a type of "perfume" made from a violet, ornamental flower that grows on a grey-green, crumbly-leaved, hairy, aromatic shrub which grows in Italy and Greece. Lavender was used in the kitchen to refine dishes such as fish, poultry, or lamb. Lavender was also used as a pleasant fragrance. Charles the Great, crowned Emperor in Rome in 800 A.D., issued an order which regulated the cultivation of the lavender shrub for use in medicine and cooking. Well-being and health went hand in hand with this shrub.

But, apart from the famous lavender water, perfumes were mostly unknown in our latitudes. The Crusaders were amazed to discover the numerous, novel "perfumes" and odors surrounding them in the Middle East. There even existed a whole, highly lucrative branch of business in the Orient devoted to the stuff. Some traders and shopkeepers concerned themselves with nothing but the secret recipes of these perfumes and other delights. Europe suddenly discovered new herbs, spices, flowers, and plants. So, with the Crusades, the fragrances spread into the West.

Venice was the main transshipment center but, also, via Egypt, Syria, Greece, and other centers in Italy, perfumes certainly entered the other countries of Europe. In France, particularly, the new perfumes and fragrances were met with great interest. Astute French merchants began to realize the golden treasure that they had accidentally encountered. With this, the trade of perfumes increased in size, especially in polite society, which saw an opportunity to be enriched with beautiful scents which they did not want to miss.

Catherine of Medici (1519–1589) was a descendant of the influential Florentine family of the Medici, who was once described as "richer than God." By her marriage to Henry II, she had landed on the French throne. She determined much of

France's fate after her husband died and her children came of age. Perhaps she had known perfumes in the Italy of her youth, which had the most direct connection with the Near East.

She is credited with introducing the sidesaddle for ladylike riding and was also regarded as the mother of French cooking. In any case, she inspired the French nobility to use special spices and ingredients. This made for a smooth transition into the use of fragrances.

In 1580, we encounter, under her rule, a highly interesting and mysterious figure – the alchemist and pharmacist Francesco Tombarelli. Alchemists enjoyed an extraordinary reputation at the time. Their goal was not only the conversion of base metals to gold and silver, but they also experimented with all kinds of substances. In those days, they had already developed distillation and extraction equipment. Sometimes, in their laboratories was an object called a "Witch's Cauldron." It boiled, steamed, and hissed. Everything was mixed and tested, under great secrecy. It was German alchemists, in many ways the first chemists, who finally discovered in 1708 the basis for porcelain*, or "white gold," as it was also called. And alchemists were not immune to the lure of profit. At least one of the co-inventors of porcelain had spent years searching for the secret of real, yellow gold. They also discovered gunpowder[1].

---

1 For completeness and historical accuracy, however, one must add that both porcelain and black powder had already been known in China for hundreds of years.

The Fatal Mutation (Part 1)

More important, however, was the fact that, with the knowledge of chemistry, artificial, chemically produced perfumes were slowly but surely making their way into everyday society. Previously, the ancient Egyptians and ancient Indians, the Greeks and Romans had used natural substances when they wanted to overpower a bad odor. Suddenly, however, all sorts of materials were being blended. And so toxic substances were also found in the following centuries in perfumes, whose first European center was the city of Grasse.

Grasse was initially an insignificant town at the southernmost tip of France, close to Italy. However, it suddenly grew to immense importance when the alchemist Tombarelli settled there. Today, Grasse is regarded as the world capital of perfume.

Many tanners made their home in Grasse. They were tradesmen, who created unpleasant odors from the leather-tanning process, and these odors needed correction.

The necessary anti-odor fragrances were at first only distilled from jasmine and orange blossoms. About 1600, these were employed initially to perfume leather gloves. But soon their side business became their primary business. Here was a completely new enterprise – money and gold in abundance. Life was glorious!

Today, flowers and necessary materials for the perfumes are imported from all parts of the world, especially from low-cost countries such as Morocco, Bulgaria, India, or Turkey. Even in those far-off days, Grasse was feverishly considering how to reduce the cost of producing its perfumes. Furthermore, in the following centuries came the discoveries of "perfuming" dishwashing detergents, washing powder and food to provide them with pleasant scents. Today, there are thirty perfume factories in Grasse.

The alchemist and pharmacist Tombarelli had opened the door to a billion-dollar industry.

Gifted with a remarkable business sense, Tombarelli initially distinguished strictly between ordinary people and the nobility. "To put good myrrh into the mouth is not for the simple man," he told those around him.[5] And so, he distinguished between "royal perfumes" and perfumes for the ordinary citizen, the bourgeoisie.

Perfumes were used in previous centuries to disinfect the air. They were considered an essential weapon in the fight against some diseases, while much later they were found to be responsible for diseases. Harmful germs were thought to be driven away by certain perfumes. As a result, the use of Eau-de-toilette became more and more fashionable.

Perfumes spread rapidly in France. But how did the perfumes come to the rest of Europe, amongst other things?

The Superior Influence of France

Let us first reiterate the point. In antiquity, "perfumes" were made exclusively from natural substances, primarily from plants. However, the mass production of perfumes from constituents free of artificial chemicals finally ended as early as the seventeenth or eighteenth century – more precisely, in France and, as we now know, even more precisely, in Grasse.

Suddenly, the production of artificial-chemical perfumes was the center of interest! At any rate, during the eighteenth, nineteenth and twentieth centuries, not to mention our twenty-first century, all at once "perfumeries" sprouted like mushrooms in the soil of almost every country.

What happened? Well, for one thing, the era of Louis XIV (1638–1715), the Sun King, contributed significantly to the spread of perfumes.

Let us not forget: In France, an entirely new level of courtly behavior had suddenly become fashionable and chic. Previously, the aristocrats had had at their disposal only a few "scratch-brushes," with which they attacked their backs so that bugs were crushed while at the same time they were skillfully conversing with the ladies. One did not shower, one bathed – some in bathing suits – and only occasionally.

In short, hygiene conditions were a pure catastrophe. There were no water closets, as we know them today. The bathing culture was at a miserable level all over Europe, except Germany. In

Germany, cleanliness was written up as virtuous. In France, one had to put up with bad odors – body odors, as well as toilet odors – and with the attempts of perfume to counteract the bad smells!

The highly refined, cultivated conduct and manners of the Sun King spread all over Europe, to all princely and royal houses, and with them did spread the *perfumes.*

But why were the French so successful in the export of their culture (one could ask in all naiveté)? Let us remember, in the seventeenth century; French was the language of scholars and educated people. First in the twelfth, thirteenth and fourteenth centuries, but still more widespread in the sixteenth, seventeenth and partly in the eighteenth century, French overtook the German and English tongue.

In the twelfth to fourteenth centuries, (French) chivalry was responsible for courtly culture, which was "fashion" and was regarded as the highest ideal that could be achieved. Throughout Europe, an attempt was made to copy this courtly culture with its chivalry – until Miguel de Cervantes (1547–1616), the best-known of all Spanish writers, made famous by his work "*Don Quixote*," in which he killed the concept of chivalry by making it seem ridiculous.

Later, the French cultural influence experienced another upsurge from the great French kings. Again, everything French became chic. Everyone who was "educated," who held some position, spoke French in the seventeenth and eighteenth centuries. This was because Louis XIV was regarded as the epitome of European leadership through his elegance and his uniquely polite manners. He also convinced others through the shining sword, for no one was militarily as successful as the Sun King during the first half of his reign. And France was the most prosperous nation on the European continent. And power seduces others to bow down before its language.

Today we use many expressions originally from French, which we believe are "English." German was similarly infiltrated by French. Let us think only of these words which are indirectly related to perfume or which at least responded to the fact that the perfume culture fell on fertile soil:

- Adventure (French: *adventure*)
- Champagne
- Diplomat (*diplomate*)
- Wardrobe (*garderobe*, meaning a coatrack)
- Jewel (*joel*)
- Mannequin (*mannequin)*
- Memoirs (*mémoires*)
- Palace (*palais*)
- Powder (*poudre*)
- Dance (*dance*)

The *savoir-faire* of food, culture, arts, fashion, and the "right" way to deal with the ladies was mainly developed in France! Once again, the French were far ahead of all other nations in the art of the seduction of women.

And so, English, Germans, Spanish and other nations borrowed their many expressions. Thousands of words were introduced, but today we hardly remember their French origin.

France and Perfume

In this way, French culture, including *perfume*, experienced tremendous expansion. Suddenly these "fragrances" were everywhere!

Louis XIV was, no doubt, a vain peacock. Some historical peasants assure us that he seduced over 2,000 women into the royal bed. This figure surpassed even Casanova's conquests. The King became a role-model, with each prince trying to copy him. The princes, in turn, were copied by the subjects. The mass use of perfumes and fragrances spread to all sections of society.

The Fatal Mutation (Part 2)

Chemists always had their hands in the game. Let us not forget that from a specific point in time, chemistry began to erode alchemy. Even the great Isaac Newton, one of the indisputable geniuses of mankind's history, a highly rational individual, attempted to trace the mystery of making gold in the eighteenth century. But these times were irrevocably over. During many experiments in the still medieval-looking laboratories, with all their crucibles, pots, glasses, and bellied glass vessels, in which things hissed, steamed, and boiled, one came closer to the trail of the secrets of chemistry.

The old, dusty doctrine of the four elements – fire, water, air, and earth – was buried in the seventeenth century, and with it, alchemy. *Chemistry* saw the light of day. One element after another was discovered. To date, our chemists know 118 elements – in contrast with only four elements of the alchemists. The new elements were arranged in the so-called "periodic table." A variety of combinations were suddenly possible. The outcome of this was an almost infinite number of chemically producible perfumes.

Various elements were joined together. Liquids, crystals, even gases were mixed, with numerous systematic and unsystematic experiments undertaken. In this turbulent atmosphere, a few chemically gifted people suddenly recognized that a cheaper way of producing fragrances was by doing so artificially. Thus, they experimented more and more with artificial, toxic substances.

In the seventeenth and eighteenth centuries, wealth was vested in the upper classes, the aristocrats and royalty. There were plenty of ladies and gentlemen whose only sport was to pursue the opposite sex, not only with the most outrageously fashionable clothes – all the buckles, gold and silver buttons, the expensive fabrics and the tailor-made ribbons – but also with new and unusual fragrances.

Those who smelt bad had no chance of impressing the opposite sex. It was apparent to the chemist that, for a long time,

money could be made in those circles, and since the aristocrats of the sixteenth, seventeenth, and eighteenth centuries
were chiefly engaged in the courting of ladies, the business
of perfumes continued to flourish. The aristocratic ladies also
saw an opportunity for attracting admirers using good perfumes.

Thus, there was a huge demand, as the economists would call
it. And so, many smart chemists took to the market to make
their riches.

When the French Revolution in 1789 finally brought the King
to the guillotine and "shortened" his reign, the power of the
aristocracy was reduced across Europe. A new target group
came into view, the aspiring middle classes, and the *nouveau
riche*, the "New Rich." The chemist, however, was indifferent
as to whose money he pulled out of whose pocket. On the contrary, the more customers who demanded perfumes, the better
the chemist's businesses succeeded.

In the early days, people were able to distinguish between different diluent (that which dilutes) classes – the scent intensity
and the scent notes. After all, the chemist wanted to use every
possible aroma: *floral, feminine, masculine, oriental, fruity,
citrus-fresh,* and *classic-elegant* fragrances.

The skillful advertiser suddenly began to play an important
role. With perfume, one proved "individuality." It purported
to show that one had "style" and "elegance." A huge attraction to the opposite sex could be exercised with perfumes

while, equally, certain perfumes allegedly made the other sex irresistible.

And today?

Around 60% of all women aged fourteen and over and 35% of all men have already used perfumes. For women over eighteen, the rate is almost 100%.

"Wait a minute," thought an advertising psychologist of the perfume industry in the early part of this century. "If we can lead 60% of all women to perfumes, why not 60% of all men? That should double our billions."

So now, men too were bombarded with perfume advertising. Concerning them, these advertising boys were excellent! With the help of advertising icons such as David Beckham and Boris Becker, today hardly any male teenager believes that he can manage without perfume.

As an aside: when I participated in a small football tournament on the fiftieth anniversary of my old home club in 2008, the place smelled worse than a hairdressing salon in the changing room and shower. In "my time," thirty years earlier, these odors did not exist.

Currently, there are about 1,100 fragrances available in stores. Each year approximately 200 new ones are added, while some old ones disappear from the market. And each fragrance contains thousands of chemicals. It is a gigantic, multi-billion-dollar business, because fragrances, highly toxic in part, are not only contained in bottled perfumes. I will cover locations where fragrances exist in abundance in a forthcoming chapter.

Perfumes containing chemical poisons were produced in large quantities during the modern era. Artificial substances saved costs and increased profits. Many chemical and synthetic substances contained oil and waste products from the oil industry, which also caused immense health damage. Poisons replaced nature; chemical mixtures replaced natural blossom fragrances. Toxins and more toxins flooded the markets.

The chemist, the brewer, the poison blender, was suddenly in favor as never before. Organic, but expensive natural substances were replaced by cheap chemicals. The complex aromas of flowers, plants, and trees were divided into their individual components. Chemists found out which elements were responsible for the fragrances, copied them chemically, and produced them artificially.

As mentioned, partially cheap, dirty, waste materials were used, all highly toxic substances. As it was "only" to sell the customer a fragrance, they felt the massive profit was justified.

Health? "Who gives a ..." was the attitude of this type of "chemist."

And this still seems to be the case today.

And what about our governments? Our Health Offices?

Is it not their responsibility to protect their citizens? One would assume so. But all I discovered over the past twenty years was that a well-hidden warning on the website of the Environmental Bureau was not even from the Ministry of Health. Apparently, the Ministry of Health ignores the danger. They seem to justify it by the fact that fragrances are emissions and therefore belong to the Environmental Agency.

There are some enlightening texts and some laws, proving that the facts about the health damage are known – but that's about all the government has done. The perfume industry laughs about it. The laws and regulations are about as useful as the net of a soccer goal when you're trying to catch herring!

More on this in a later chapter. Back to history, to the triumphal march of perfume:

The trend was unstoppable.

But who turned the wheels behind the scenes? "Priests," alchemists and pharmacists were just a small part of the unholy alliance. Soon another group joined the plan, which one must understand if one wants to comprehend how the spread of the perfume industry continued.

The Psychologist

In the twentieth century, if not before, it was discovered that one could sell just about anything with fragrances. Clothes could be perfumed, toys, detergents – I will explain point by point in the next chapter exactly how the global spread of highly toxic perfumes occurred.

Hundreds of services and thousands of goods could be sold more effectively, the so-called "advertising psychologist" suggested to the dealers, suppliers, and producers.

All they had to do was add fragrance. Huge markets could be rapidly acquired. Millions of additional dollars could be made by attracting customers with scented products.

Recall the so-called Brahmin "priests" who earlier incited their "customers" with incense and similar fragrances!

At this point, a small confession. In my childhood and youth, I felt drawn to pleasing aromas. Ah, that incense! The church always smelt so good. The incense flowed from a vessel which was oh-so-beautifully swung back and forth by my brother – at that time an altar-boy. *That's* why I always looked for a place very close to the front pew. Our priest ever considered me a particularly good Christian. Hm, hm, hm?

Let's remain with the theme of "money and perfume."

At the words of the advertising psychologist, surely the heart of every entrepreneur beat faster, excitedly, with the idea of conquering new markets. It was music to his ears. New markets? Ha! – that was what he had always been waiting for!

The advertising psychologist (including other psychologists and psychiatrists) – we shall call each and all a "psych" for the sake of simplicity because in America it is now a common term – suddenly began to spray their poisonous ideas everywhere. Their insinuations were believed – "Well-being, sex, huge profits, and expansion." That was it!

This was the ne-plus-ultra of the seller's new reality. The seed was planted in the entire economy. With secret odors, according to the psychologist, one could increase turnover enormously, at incredible speed. The psych whispered to the entrepreneur, from the simple supermarket to the largest hotel chains and airlines, that one could fool the customer in this respect.

Using fragrances and perfumes, he or she would be prevented from differentiating between one product and another and so could not come to any objective judgment. Customers let themselves be manipulated magnificently. They could be seduced in the literal sense. Senses could be fogged to encourage them to buy. Wonderful world! You just have to pretend that something smells very good and you could pull the consumer like a donkey by its nose ring to make more and more purchases.

This "advertising psychology" was suddenly very busy. The psychologist, the great manipulator, became the closest ally of the chemist and perfumeries. An uncanny covenant was created here, to the exclusion of the public. Thus, synthetic[1] perfumes, with their terrible side effects, began to spread rapidly, but under the guise of pleasant scents.

Even food is "perfumed" today with artificial flavors and smells, just to allow people to be coaxed into making more purchases. Anything that *can* be perfumed *is* perfumed. This includes household goods of all kinds, clothes, even cars. Yes, even in vehicles we find perfumes today! In this context, I recall a TV documentary on how perfume experts, along with advertising professionals, worked on fragrances to mask the smell of new cars, perceived as unpleasant by most customers. I would judge that as a risk to drivers, now that I am aware that perfume chemicals can cause a reduction in one's alertness.

There is much more to this topic.

To make you feel comfortable when you travel, you are sprayed with chemicals (disinfectants and perfumes) in airplanes from numerous air nozzles. On a flight from Dubai to Frankfurt, I woke up in an Emirate Airlines aircraft with a sneezing fit. My airways seemed to be full of these chemicals in the truest

------

1 The words "synthetic", "artificial", and "chemical" are synonymous (meaning the same). So are the words "natural" and "organic." It is this very type of perfume, the synthetic perfume = the artificial perfume = the chemical perfume, that is the very opposite of natural perfume = organic perfume.

sense of the word. My body reacted. I was not the only one to do so. In my seating area, there were at least three other people who had to sneeze four to six times.

More and more, one realizes that many passengers, especially after long-haul flights, have health problems. The state's "experts" point fingers at the dry air that prevails in airplanes. My God, how stupid! Dry air you can endure for days, even weeks, without problems.

There is still more that I would call perfume traps.

Travel with your children into London to Hamley's, the toy-shopping paradise. A wall of sweet perfume is waiting for you at the entrance. It is as if you were bumping against a solid glass barrier. Your children will ignore this because, at this moment, their attention is only on the colorful world of toys. The runny nose, the cough, wheezing or similar reactions may not occur until days later.

There is even more.

Have you ever been sick from a holiday or a business trip lasting several days? The advertising psychs have conquered not only the men's and women's and children's worlds but also all international hotel chains and almost all other accommodation outlets in the last ten years. Already, in the hotel lobby, today's visitor is usually hit in the face with a cloud of perfume.

In four- and five-star hotels, everything is perfumed: from the lobby to the towel to the bed linen. For a long time, three-star hotels were relatively safe. But recently this dream came to an end in Brazil, in a city about fifty km north of Sao Paulo. Perhaps it was just a two-star hotel, but it smelled penetratingly of six stars!

Therefore, I am happy every time my business leads me to China. This is almost a secret tip for travelers. Check out Chinese hotels in China. They are perfume-free! At least this was still true in 2015. But beware: hotels which belong to international Western chains are still perfumed even in China.

Flying in China is also pleasant. None of the passengers and flight attendants are perfumed there. But flights *to* China are, on the other hand, the usual horror. Almost every non-Chinese passenger has some eau-de-toilette on the skin or a "chemical laboratory under the armpit," as Dr. Mauch calls it so aptly in his book, *Die Bombe unter der Achselhöhle* (The Armpit Bomb).

It seems as if the psychs have not yet conquered China. I love my China! (This is an allusion to the beautiful song by Song Zuying, "我 我 中 国").

This is not even everything, though.

Just think of perfumed baby clothes. For heaven's sake, dear mothers! What newborn babies need, with their still-very-fragile cells, is fresh, clean air! Don't get me wrong – the mistakes that are made here are not to be blamed on the mothers — the finger points to advertising psychologists, perfume manufacturers, and chemical manufacturers.

I would not be surprised if it turns out that the high infant mortality rates in various hospitals are attributable to the delusion of a hygienic, healthy environment created by (often-overdone) disinfectant chemicals and perfumed rooms with perfumed bedding.

But let's stick to the facts. We cannot prove that now.

No one has pointed out to this day the extent to which the customer of perfume is deceived and pays not only with his money but also with his health. He does not always pay immediately, but ultimately, he pays with premature death, according to prestigious critics of perfumes, whom I will quote later in more detail.

But before I spread more "bad news," we should first allow ourselves an interim summary.

Interim Summary

It is a surprise to realize that three types of people have pushed for the triumph of perfumes. The devious "priest," the "chemist" and the "psych" have all at one time, or another entered an unholy alliance, to the detriment of the consumer.

There's nothing wrong with the basic urge for procreation followed by a hunt for sex – but if sex is manipulated malignantly, is misdirected and shamelessly exploited, one must be allowed to raise a voice in protest. In any case, these three "types," especially those acting behind the scenes, insisted that the entire human race undergo the "wonderful benefits" of perfumes. They have opened a Pandora's box with their learned-sounding words, thus gifting the whole human race with poisonous fragrances – specifically, with health-damaging substances inhaled and applied to the skin.

Nowadays, numerous illnesses can unquestionably be traced back to perfumes, as I will prove. It is a very exciting and yet horrifying thriller. We never previously asked to *whom* we owe this "blessing," which is a curse – the curse of artificial perfumes.

Once again, the money-hungry "priest," the "chemist" (the poison expert) and the unscrupulous, seductive "advertising psychologist" are responsible. They have made sure that one of the greatest evils imaginable, of *poisoned air to breathe*, has been inflicted upon Mankind.

Let us take a deep breath, hopefully of fresh air, and stop for a moment. Only by realizing what is going on with the perfume industry, we have already understood a great deal. We have identified the manipulators and the puppet masters. Yet, we still do not know precisely to what *degree* perfumes have been infiltrated into society. We still do not know the full truth. In the twentieth and twenty-first centuries, perfumes were, in a variety of ways, pushed through the back door into many sectors, markets and countries that were unaware of what damage they were doing. It has been part of a planned conquest of the entire planet Earth, including an insidious conquest of our olfactory nerves.

Let us consider this conquest, which has so far escaped the attention of the public, and in detail continue to reveal this secret, hidden, well-covered trail of the psychs.

Define the terms!

VOLTAIRE
French writer and philosopher (1694–1778)

CHAPTER 3

A Treacherous Definition

I HAVE ALREADY pointed out that perfumes, containing devastating poisons, are now to be found everywhere, even on distant mountain farms in Chechnya. But wait a moment! Before we draw attention to its worldwide distribution, we must first introduce a precise definition of the word "perfume." In this context, we can look forward to a surprise!

To get to the bottom of an understanding of perfumes, we should first of all look at some dictionaries, so that we can get a good idea of what the word "perfume" actually means. (Please note: the following references are to German dictionaries. You may find it interesting to see whether the definition of perfume is the same in an English dictionary.)

According to *Duden* (2005), a dictionary that the high-school teacher Konrad Duden once composed to improve the spelling of his pupils, a perfume is an:

> *"alcoholic liquid, in which fragrances are dissolved;* also, a *liquid with an intense, long-lasting smell"*

The dictionary called *Wahrig* (2005), written by Professor Wahrig, affirms that a perfume is:

> *"A mostly aqueous-alcoholic solution of animal or synthetic, but predominantly vegetable-origin odoriferous substances."*

Aha! The *Wahrig* is, therefore, somewhat more precise; it already points to the *synthetic,* that is, the *artificial, chemical* odoriferous substances. But we still do not know precisely what perfumes are.

However, why should you have to work through all these definitions with your mind? After all, they are defining real, observable items. So, why shouldn't you clarify some facts with your senses – with your nose, for example? Let us make an attempt. Have a go with a little test.

Experiment: Flowers vs Perfume

Immerse your head in a big bouquet of fresh flowers and breathe in deeply ten times! Take ten deep breaths, so that air penetrates to the farthest corners of your lungs.

Then ask yourself the question, how do you feel?

Of course, you will feel *fantastic*; nothing is more refreshing than a natural, pleasant smell, especially the smell of a fresh bouquet.

WARNING:

Only do the following experiment if you are in good, stable health. If you have a condition relating to asthma, the heart, or circulatory weaknesses, then this test could be harmful to you.

Grab two perfume bottles and open them. Hold an opening to each nostril. Take ten deep breaths through your nose and allow the smell to penetrate through the nose to the lungs.

Now ask yourself the question, how do you feel?

Ah, there is a certain discomfort? Maybe a headache? Very interesting!

If that happens, I can only congratulate you. Your natural defense systems still work excellently. Your body defends itself against the perfume toxins and gives you (painful) warning signals. You could say your instinct warns you against perfumes.

So, you can also define the term *"perfume"* by the nose. And perfumes are almost always poisonous. Artificial. Chemical. Approximately 99.9% of all perfumes contain the type of chemical substances for which you can read "poisons."

But let's go further through the thicket of definitions, as it becomes more and more interesting.

Browse the Internet, search for what the "online encyclopedia" *Wikipedia* describes.

Wikipedia? The made-up word is composed of *Wiki* (= Hawaiian: *fast*) and *pedaia* (= Greek: *education*). Aha! So, *Wikipedia* gives us a "quick education." This is what we need now. What do the Wikipedians teach us? Oh, the friends and experts there lay it out!

They tell us that fragrances are odors, odor mixtures and odor compositions that *"change or mask body odor."* They also tell us that room scents are *"perfumes laced with special odors ... directly through sprays ..."*

And then it becomes revealing. According to (the German) *Wikipedia* (in other languages it might read differently):

Perfumes are also:

> *"odors that are supposed to make a variety of products attractive for the consumer ... Many products in the bathroom, kitchen, house, and garden are perfumed ... such as detergents or hair dyes. [They] are made pleasant to the buyer with fragrances ..."*[1]

As to *perfume*s in the broadest sense, meaning "aromas," this is a specialized area, which I would not want to get involved with here. "Aroma" has more to do with the topic of food and drink. Breathing, drinking, and eating are three basic needs of man. This book, however, is dedicated primarily only to breathing.

We should also mention here the principle of tiny (but poisonous) quantities which are *supposed* to be harmless. We do know examples from history, where kings and popes systematically poisoned their bodies so that the organism could slowly get used to it. They typically took minute amounts of arsenic and increased the amount a little each day. In the event of a real arsenic attack, the body was already adjusted to the poison, and so it would no longer be fatal. In this way, assassins could be beaten. How much such an act harms one, however, is another question. I would not advise anyone to perform such a foolish "security measure." Moreover, arsenic is an exceptional case. In the case of most poisons, humans cannot build up a tolerance in this way.

A body has amazing defense mechanisms. To some extent, it even can survive many unhealthy items, even poisons. But every load has its limit. Too many different toxins, or even regularly lower doses of a single toxin, or mixtures of toxins that can be tolerated on their own but become harmful in combination, can reach this limit.

But, you say, in the case of the tiny doses involved with perfume, surely an organism would have to be subjected to dozens or even hundreds of such poisons during the same period for there to be a noticeably harmful effect.

Do you want to hear the truth? The bare facts?

3,000 to 5,000 different chemicals are now found in perfumes!

Over 80% of them were never tested for adverse reactions on humans.

Sometimes, a single bottle of perfume contains several hundred different chemicals – in extreme cases, up to 400.[2]

Let us repeat: A single bottle of perfume can contain up to 400 different poisons!

Therefore, 15–30% of the population now suffers from chemical sensitivity. Children are the worst affected, but the maximum input of perfumes/chemicals is often exceeded even in adults. Most of the people concerned do not even know about this fact. They may feel uncomfortable sometimes and can hardly describe their symptoms accurately before some disease finally hits hard and mercilessly.[3]

Do you see it? It is impossible that a body today, in the twenty-first century, can withstand this onslaught of perfume poisons and "get used to" it. Every day, "beauty-conscious" women slap up to 515 chemical substances on their faces.[4] However, practically nothing is publicly known about the toxic effects, especially the long-term effects, of most perfume chemicals despite early warnings given for many years.[5]

The Naiveté of the Consumer ...

..., in short, is abused. Trustingly, customers assume that they are doing something good for themselves when they use creams, cosmetics, perfumes, and so on. They do not know that developments in the cosmetics industry have been similar to developments in the food industry.

In both cases, the market ultimately dictates the ingredients. The entrepreneur tries to reduce production costs here and there. This has meant, in plain words, that synthetic, inexpensive, often toxic substances form part of the product. Scrooge won the war – the economic war. The same is true in the cosmetics industry. Even extravagantly expensive perfumes sometimes contain regular poison bombs. Unfortunately, one cannot describe it differently if one wants to tell the truth.

Imagine this scenario: you wake up in the morning, happy and without a care, and take a shower. You use a scented soap. With a scented shampoo, you wash your hair. Then afterward you shave wet, with a shaving foam which also contains perfumes. Or you shave dry and electric, then use a scented aftershave.

You may also use a (perfumed) deodorant that you spray under the armpits. From there, through the body's circulatory systems, it reaches the entire body very quickly. Using a (perfumed) moisturizing cream, you rub some dry skin surfaces, then maybe use a (scented) body lotion.

You eat breakfast. Added aromas (and therefore perfumes) are in your morning meal.

Off to the office. The rooms have been spritzed, mopped, and wiped with cleaning agents which also contain perfumes. Furthermore, the rooms were then sprayed with perfumes *as* perfumes so that everything would "smell good." There you are, preparing for a good day's mental work, inhaling the stale, poisonous air.

Your secretary is wrapped in a single perfume cloud. Your co-workers have used different aftershaves, deodorants, soaps, shampoos, colognes. You cannot prevent yourself from re-inhaling perfumes on a massive scale.

Just like the **passive smoker**, there is also the **passive perfume sniffer**.

A second lady, another colleague, is also perfumed from head to toe and smells (frankly) like a brothel. She stops to chat. Once again, you get your portion of this poison. Everywhere, men and women alike pass you by, wafting perfumes under your nose all day long.

Your clothes, at least, are safe, have been carefully cleaned. But alas, you have forgotten that dry-cleaning also uses perfumes. Laundry fresheners are infused with perfume chemicals. Even new clothes you wear on your skin may have been treated with perfumes – to help them sell.

A small tip: Wash new clothes before their first wear with perfume-free detergents.

And on that occasion, add all your other laundry and treat it the same way because all your detergents at home are most likely perfumed, usually without you or your partner being aware of this fact.

After all, you have grown up with perfumes and have considered it completely "normal."

I think we can reflect a little here. A normal man, an average woman, lives under a perfume-cloud, whether realizing it or not, whether approving of it or not.

Now add up those vast amounts of toxins you are exposed to every day. Your body cannot possibly get rid of them all. It protests. It gives you warnings. You suddenly feel uncomfortable. But it does not change anything. Perfumes are everywhere. They spread like the Biblical plague of locusts in ancient Egypt.

The actual scenario is even more explosive — the biggest scandal I haven't yet exposed.

Perfumes and the Environment

Since we are now a friend of useful dictionaries, we should look at the word "aerosol" under the magnifying glass.

Do you have any idea of what is coming?

Tiny, invisible, solid or liquid suspended substances in gases or the air are called "aerosols."

In Latin, *aer* = *air* and *solutio* = *solution*.

Let us repeat this. It is very revealing. The term *aerosol* is used to indicate *liquid* or *solid suspended particles* which have been mixed with gas. Liquid and gaseous perfume ingredients can cause damage and disruption on the skin, in the lungs, the bloodstream and brain, but are also quite readily eliminated from the body and environment. However, as noted, aerosols can also contain a more enduring danger which matters to us. *Solid particles*! A gas can be volatile and seem to dissolve into nothingness, a liquid can evaporate and be carried away as individual molecules which will break down more or less rapidly on exposure to enzymes, oxygen, sunlight, etc., but a solid particle lasts longer. It is very "concrete," and it is spread around the environment when the gases are sprayed.

Perfumes in aerosols may contain, be carried by, or even mostly consist of these *small, solid particles*. Such particles do not evaporate rapidly. They do not disappear into nowhere. On the contrary, they remain until they are physically broken down – if, indeed, they are capable of being physically broken down by natural processes.

Confusing? Chemistry! Let me simplify what that means: the toxins of the perfumes never dissolve. Once sprayed, they will forever pollute our environment and breathing air. The scent only disappears if the perfume will have been diluted enough in the ambient air. Once sprayed, they exist on and on and on! Indestructible!

Through the air, over the atmosphere, perfumes are spread. Poison is diffused into the environment. The solid particles are carried through the air, even into the remotest places on planet Earth, to every nook and corner.

That means that we can no longer escape perfumes today, even if we know the consequences of exposure to them. We are exposed willy-nilly to these poisons, which are deliberately used in perfumes. Their liquids and gases evaporate fast and are inhaled as molecules which can interfere with the body's natural processes. The tiny, solid particles of the aerosol perfumes likewise travel through the air you breathe, but also settle in the environment, are picked up by the wind, and persist. Wherever you go, therefore, perfumes will reach you, and you will inhale them.

The particles are so tiny that they can even pass through the lungs and penetrate any part of the systems of the body. Some molecules of perfume are small enough to pass across the blood-brain barrier. Within seconds after being inhaled, these poisons reach the brain and any other cell in your body. And so, we suffer all kinds of hard-to-treat illnesses, ranging from the simple headache to "inexplicable" allergies, to cancer – diseases with unknown, unknowable, or multiple causes or.

The body needs clean, fresh air to stay healthy. Only then does it live well.

The more corrupt the air, the more the lungs are infected with poisons which reach into the whole bodily system, and the more easily it becomes diseased.

Usually, we can perceive poisons with the nose. The instinctive warning system which we all possess warns us, for example, that "something stinks!" But precisely because this warning system is overridden by perfumes – because they "smell so good" – we fail to notice the danger signals!

Self-Destruction

We should be shocked to discover that, by inhaling perfumes, we are slowly but surely building up a poisonous deposit that makes us secretly but certainly ill. Since perfume "smells good," smells excellent, we tolerate it. In this way, we slowly sniff ourselves into various diseases. The toxic chemicals get into the lungs, the brain, the blood, and finally, our entire bodily system.

Perfumes – let's end this fallacy finally – do not have anything to do with hygiene. Soap cleanses. Pure alcohol cleanses. Perfumes never cleanse. Perfumes do not have the slightest detergent or cleaning power.

And so, just from examining a few definitions, we can immediately see that we find ourselves today surrounded by and exposed to myriad perfumes or, rather, toxins that we cannot escape. And we cannot escape from these toxins even if we resent and dislike them, and even if we are more enlightened than our peers about the risks, they pose to our well-being and health.

Women in the so-called "highly developed" countries are the first and primary victims of perfumes, owing to false and misleading cosmetics commercials. Their minds are conditioned day after day, year after year, with incorrect ideas and information. It is nothing better than subtle brainwashing by advertising psychologists. Women, primarily, are the people being manipulated into believing that they need perfume so they can smell good and look good – or even just "acceptable."

The truth is that perfumes are toxins that make you sick. Through women, who are very often the opinion-leaders of the family and community in terms of hygiene, beauty, and health, the artificial and false "need" for perfumes created by advertisers also permeates the lives and awareness of children and men.

And so, suddenly and somewhat surprisingly, we can begin to perceive the pitfalls that surround perfumes. These are pitfalls into which we can all too easily tumble. We are exposed to them at every turn of our aromatic world.

This is only a humble beginning. I have so far only innocently presented some definitions. I have not yet explained where perfumes are already being used today. I have merely picked up the scent!

All secrets remain so only for a particular time.

KRISTINA OF SWEDEN
Queen of Sweden and Duchess of Bremen-Verden (1626–1689)

CHAPTER 4

Omnipresent Perfumes and Poisons

AFTER ALL THE above, we now know in which direction we must look when it comes to perfumes and poisons. We have taken a huge step in the right direction.

In addition, although we cannot avoid perfumes, several concrete remedies already exist. I will introduce these in detail, beginning with some at the end of this chapter. Nothing is impossible. You can recover your health. One can poison a body 100% and completely detoxify it 100%. But first, we must understand the full extent of the poisoning intellectually and have all the information. Only then can we strike back effectively and quickly.

In this chapter, we will reveal several more surprises. For that purpose, let's follow the day-to-day routine of a twenty-five-year-old woman. And let's call this modern-day Cinderella "Cindy."

Cindy is unmarried, and she is looking for a man – an appropriate "soulmate," as it is so aptly worded these days. Perhaps she might even be a candidate for marriage, although she would never admit it. She is intelligent, attractive, and well-endowed by Mother Nature and selective about partners. She works in a computer company and keeps fit, often going hiking, and exercising regularly in a fitness center. Also, Cindy loves her little nephew, her sister's son.

So, what is her daily routine?

The Morning Poisons

No sooner has Cindy woken up, stretched, and yawned than she runs to the bathroom. As she pays attention to cleanliness and well-being, she has toilet-rim blocks to perfume and color the water in the toilet. She also has a fragrance dispenser mounted on the cistern. "Good smells." On the day that she finds the right man, she is determined that he should be immediately impressed by the "wonderful smells" in her environment.

As early as 1985, researchers were asking whether there was such a thing as an illness caused by air fresheners. The lack of awareness in the general population that such a phenomenon is possible can be explained in part by a countervailing tide of advertisement and lobbying to normalize perfume use and prevent health concerns from becoming more widely talked about.[1]

Cindy is inspired in this thinking by her external surround-ings because practically every public toilet today has such a fragrance dispenser; even in hospitals, schools, and so on, the scent makes things *seem* more hygienic.

But wait! Cindy has no idea that even seemingly harmless toilet-rim blocks and the toilet fragrance dispenser can con-tain perfume poisons. These are the first things that Cindy breathes after waking up: poisons!

⋆⫵ ⫴⋆

Only for the expert
and those who want to know exactly

Toilet blocks often contain, among other chemicals: acetone, ethanol and acetaldehyde, toxic substances.
Octanal, 3-hexene-1-ol, ethanol, pinenes, nonanal, linalool and d-limonene have been found in toilet dispensers.
Scientists have unequivocally established this fact.[2]

⋆⫵ ⫴⋆

Cindy, as it happens, is quite health-conscious, and had care-fully studied the product information for her perfumed prod-ucts. On the product packaging and "safety data sheets," however, she had *not* been informed about these particular poisons.

A word on "safety data sheets," a laughable title. Cindy was merely informed that the perfume ingredients were "trade secrets." How convenient! This allows the inclusion of all possible poisons which happen to be perfumes to be swept under the carpet.

Do you see how the consumer is hoodwinked?

We know there are similar tricks in the arms trade. To cover up all kinds of goings-on, it is stated that "for reasons of security" no information can be given. Under this cover, the most incredible deals take place – billion-dollar deals.

As far as toxic substances are concerned, too, we are fooled. We are not enlightened.

Now Cindy gets into the shower. She's a simple girl who uses soap, shampoo, and conditioner.

Let's assume that she uses an unperfumed soap. That's great! But as Cindy turns to her hair, she has no idea that more than 2,500 different substances are used to achieve the "correct aroma" for shampoos.

In other words, most shampoos are the wildest chemical creations. And it is rare for the customer to discover what substances are contained in such a product accurately. Why?

The European Union, theoretically the most zealous watchdog on behalf of the individual, allows manufacturers to indicate merely "perfume" in their lists of ingredients. Behind this simple word, however, everything can be hidden. "Perfume," according to the EU, does not need to be broken down into its component substances on the label. It can include *any number* of component substances, none of which needs be declared.

Here, too, it is said to be a "trade secret." A large proportion of shampoos, therefore, contain "sales-promoting fragrance components," including poisons. Scientists have managed to establish that.[3] But, just as with the air fresheners, most of the health-threatening fragrances and ingredients in shampoos cannot be identified from the published list of ingredients. Even a cautious, somewhat pedantic person, who carefully studies and reads the small print to inform himself of potentially toxic ingredients, is hopelessly misled.

Allergies and some diseases are often triggered by shampoos – more of that later.

"But why are we so misguided?" you may ask. "Do we not live in the 'best of all possible worlds,' as some philosopher ironically once called our time? Do our politicians not have among other things, a duty to protect our health?"

Well, yes, in theory, this is correct. But in practice, it is about money. The chemical industry plays hardball. The lobbyists in Brussels and Washington try everything, and I mean *everything*, to prevent their products from being banned. Today, manufacturers are allowed to refer to perfumes ("aroma" =

"perfume" = "fragrance" = "scent"), without having to separate the individual components more precisely.

Did you know that the ratio between pharma-lobbyists and Congressmen in the US is two to one? Do you know how close the interdependencies are between politics and the economy? Not infrequently, the representatives elected by the people for a few years (i.e., politicians) have no expert knowledge of the portfolio over which they suddenly reign as ministers. The result? They get information from their "consultants," who are, guess who? The lobbyists!

Back to Cindy and **Morning Poisons**:

And so, Cindy is, in good faith, washing her long, beautiful, blond hair with a shampoo containing poisons. She will then coat it with a conditioner containing its own perfume cocktail. Many shampoos and conditioners are bought primarily for the attraction of their scent, which has nothing to do with their washing and conditioning power. The magazine *Öko-Test* (a German environmental publication) has shown in studies that more than 60% of their tested shampoos contained *synthetic musk perfumes*, which can cause cancer.[4]

'Musk,' here, refers to the strong-smelling product of anal glands in certain species including the musk deer, which is so called because it possesses such glands. Another species which has been hunted for these glandular products is the civet cat. Musk has a very animal smell, but it also 'fixes' other scent molecules so that a perfume doesn't evaporate so quickly, and therefore it has been an essential ingredient in perfumes. Synthetic musk performs the same job but doesn't smell so animal-like, and isn't so hard on the species which are otherwise hunted down but synthetic musk has been implicated as a significant health hazard, too.[5]

In about a quarter of the shampoos examined by the same magazine, formaldehyde was also found. Formaldehyde is a colorless gas at room temperature with a pungent smell. It can cause allergies and irritation to the respiratory tract, skin, and eyes. In high concentrations, it affects memory, the ability to concentrate, and sleep.[6]

But oh, Cindy has only just begun to cover herself with morning poison. It goes on. She brushes her teeth, moisturizes, and makes herself up. A small (poison) thriller could be written about:

- Toothpaste
- Lipsticks and lip-liners
- Skin creams (the mix of harmful substances can be considerable)[7]
- Anti-aging creams
- Body lotions
- Eyeliners, eyeshadows, brow-liners, mascaras
- Deodorants (against body odor)
- Antiperspirants (against sweating)
- Dry shampoos, anti-frizz sprays, 'sleeking' products, heat protection …
- Waxing strips and depilatory creams

We must also include perfumes in products that are poured on or sprayed as well as brushed, smeared, or powdered. And for the gentlemen, let us not forget

- shaving foams
- aftershave
- beard oils
- hair gels, etc.,
as well as their
- share of the products above.

Books could be filled on every single heading above because there are perfumed, poisonous substances everywhere which are regularly deposited on unsuspecting consumers.

Although there are state institutions in many countries that are supposed to protect us from harm, the testers hardly succeed in documenting even the existence of these substances. In every new product that is praised as the best thing since sliced bread, there are frequently numerous chemical compounds which can only be examined with considerable effort and at a high cost.[8]

I want to define a new concept, the *criminal product*. Definition: criminal products are products that are designed with some certain knowledge or even the deliberate intention that they will harm end-users. Please do not go on believing that the manufacturers of such products do not know what they are doing.

Examples are:

- Street drugs
- Psychotropic drugs that are supposed to "help" against invented "diseases," but have devastating side effects
- Fertilizers, pesticides or herbicides that leave behind substances that are harmful to health in food and soil, and which poison the water supply for the plant and animal world
- Landmines
- Chemical weapons
- Nuclear weapons
- Biological weapons
- Chemically produced perfumes.

Any government that allows or even encourages criminal products is as criminal as the product it allows.

But back to the subject of perfumes.

These are the hard facts. Even young girls already use up to thirteen different beauty products in a day, each of which may contain twenty or more different components.[9]

Women like our pretty Cindy use even more products. "Beauty-conscious" women will rub up to 515 chemicals onto their face, every day, as mentioned. This leaves a bitter taste in one's mouth.

No human being, no institute, can test all these products, which are also regularly updated. The perfume industry laughs at regulations. Once it has been caught out, a product that has entered the headlines for its adverse effects on health will be replaced by another one.

This new "wonderful" product then sees the light of day and the perfume-maker rubs his hands at the expense of the consumer's health.

Perfume industry bosses must be thinking along these lines:

"So, now the opposition, those darned eco-testers, must once again get to work doing the research and testing to catch up to us! Let them grind their teeth, these health freaks. Let them spend enormous sums on complicated, protracted cases. For as long as the delays can be stretched out, our money-making can continue!"

Also, the perfume industry's counterarguments can now be launched in the press, i.e., positive statements about their perfume products. But if a magazine article exposing negative facts about perfume is not 100% accurate, it is attacked with complex and convoluted complaints.

The "power of the press" is often used to put testers and scientists (mostly toxicologists) on the defensive when they issue warnings about perfumes. Using *black propaganda*, as the expert calls it, more than one "enemy" of the perfume industry has been slaughtered who could have sounded the alarm.

Morning Poisons: Third Part

There is a feast of poisoning whenever bedlinen and clothes are "cleaned" with perfumed detergents. In cosmetics, approximately 8,500 different ingredients are listed that have not yet been researched. How many are found in detergents is still unclear. There are liquid detergents, fabric softeners, and fragrance products for the dryer in which toxic substances are *not even listed.*[9]

This hiding of vital data is the employment of the same old obfuscation tactics. We certainly know that there are numerous poisons in different detergents, but where and how do we find the data?

In the meantime, there are fragrances for socks, shoe linings, shoe polish with "floral scents"![10] Even menstrual pads and tampons are perfumed!

So, our pretty Cindy gets dressed and of course, putting on her freshly washed clothes, conditioned with "spring fragrance" fabric softeners, she again comes into contact with numerous perfume poisons.

It is nice, as a writer, to be able to dress or undress fictional women, as and when one pleases, but it hurts to watch them poison themselves, even to weaken their immune system, make themselves sick, and thereby rapidly lose their youthful beauty and, worse, their energy, their vibrant enjoyment of life.

Our dear Cindy finally looks as though she is ready for the catwalk. She wears a smart business suit, but she does not know what she is doing to herself with her clothes – not to mention the hurried breakfast with its numerous, added "flavorings" that she is now swiftly ingesting. Cindy looks at the clock; she's late. No time to catch the subway.

That she misses her train is not at all regrettable, however, since many stations and subway stations are now sprayed with perfumes like in London.[11] Platforms and subway corridors have long been the focus of perfume experts. Lucky escape for Cindy there.

So, Cindy dashes to her automobile. She must hurry now. In her vehicle, dangling on the retaining bracket of the rear-view mirror is a "scent tree" – these are also used nowadays in nearly all taxicabs.

Oh, darn! Perfumed again! There is no place to hide!

The journal *Öko-Test* has already warned against these dangling fragrances, these small, pretty, cardboard trees, and other novelty shapes, because some of them contain seriously harmful perfumes, damaging for the liver, kidneys and even the reproductive organs – yes, you read correctly, reproductive organs.

Öko-Test warns that around half of such "scent trees" are dangerous.[12] But that does not help this time. Cindy puts her foot down, races to her workplace and parks the car in an underground parking lot, which is, thank heaven, not yet perfumed.

But the 'odor-villain' in pursuit of poor Cindy does not care. In a parking lot, there are already enough other toxins, car exhaust or fine dust, that reach the brain within seconds after inhaling – in principle, functioning just like perfumes which first numb your senses and then proceed to make you ill.

But Cindy barely enters her company building, escaping the exhaust fumes, before she is again encountering perfume odors.

Perfumes in the Workplace

Apart from the restrooms, many *offices* – the workspaces themselves – have long since been fragranced. Not only are the cleaning agents used in offices enriched with perfumes (i.e., poisons), room sprays are also used more and more.

However, room sprays can lead to health damage, especially in pregnant women and infants. This warning was reported by the *German Green Cross* in Marburg, with reference to a British study at the University of Bristol. Headaches and pregnancy-related depressions can be the effect on women, while babies can experience diarrhea and ear infections.[13]

One must keep in mind that oxygen is vital for every human organism. If necessary, we can get by from four to eight weeks without food, we can even live for five days without water, but only one to two minutes without oxygen. Automobile exhaust gases reduce the quality of the air, as do asbestos particles and dust, and then, as you might have guessed, about 99% of all perfumes. Small particles of solids, aerosols, as I have already pointed out, penetrate the airways and wreak similar damage to asbestos dust.

Cindy is now breathing in perfume (poisons) again. She cannot avoid it. Humans breathe in and out around 20,000 times a day. In most cases, the air in the room, even within your own four walls, is contaminated with many toxins. Private rooms are sometimes up to fifty times more toxic than busy traffic intersections in big cities![14] We are rarely pampered with a "poison-free" zone.

Sprays and perfumes can even affect cardiovascular health. Heart problems can occur as a result of exposure, as proven by the experts of the Tropics and Public Health Institute in Basel.[15]

Once again, the ubiquitous fragrances with their harmful chemicals are "above the law."[16] So, we do not know just what is contained in the perfume sprays that pollute the office. No safety data sheets clarify this.

Even if safety data sheets exist and you study them thoroughly, you are often frustrated by meager, incomplete information. "Fragrance" or "perfume" is all it says. What conclusion can be drawn from that? Some safety data sheets are, therefore, hopelessly incomplete in terms of toxicity.

Time and again, manufacturers hide behind the excuse of "trade secrets" or "confidential business information," which one is supposed to respect. The truth is often simply that consumers would not buy certain products if it became crystal-clear that by doing so, they are slowly but surely poisoning themselves.

A comprehensive, cost-intensive, chemical analysis is rarely financially viable. We are exposed to endless subtle dangers, invisible dangers, poisons that hide their health-damaging activities under a pleasant scent, and so we are fooled. Subliminally and unconsciously, we constantly breathe in toxins, toxins, toxins.

Cindy keeps inhaling these poisons. Quietly, around the clock, she sniffs perfumes without knowing it. Perfume pursues Cindy like an evil spirit at every step.

Even in her office, her workstation, she is not safe from poisons. *Computer Bild* (a German computer periodical) has long since clarified that harmful substances are contained in computer housings, headphones, cables and so on. 118 products were put to the test some time ago. The testers found that 100 of them were "questionable" in health terms.

⟡⟡ ⟡⟡

Only for the expert
and those who want to know exactly

Scientists found that the electrical and electronic equipment of and around the computer contained highly toxic heavy metals such as lead, chlorinated paraffin, SVHC (Substances of Very High Concern) flame retardants and dyes that are detrimental to health. Dangers arise from the additives in the plastic parts of the computer, from "plasticizers." Plastic – actually a hard, brittle material – becomes elastic only by the addition of plasticizers. These substances, however, are not safely fixed in the plastic but are gassed out over time, as the toxicologist Professor Edmund Maser of the University of Kiel noted. This results in increased breast-cancer risk, but other hormonal damages may also occur.[17]

⊷⊷ ⊷⊷

Here, to begin with, at least, we are facing an issue of harmful, breathable chemicals which probably don't smell good but are not masked with "nice-smelling-chemicals." But this issue would not be solved by spraying equipment with yet more harmful, breathable chemicals which *do* smell good. The problem would become worse, from a health point of view! But of course, it is much better from a sales point of view.

A similar problem is faced by car industries selling from Japan via Germany to the US: brand new cars stink of all kinds of unpleasant, breathable chemicals. And each car company, therefore, spends millions to make their new cars smell "new" and "good." So-called Perfume Marketing Experts have figured out scents that cover up the metallic and plastic smells with an artificial leather smell to make selling easier.[18]

Mercedes goes even one step beyond the selling point; they make sure that their cars smell "good" not only in the show-rooms but also year after year, by adding perfume into the air filter systems in their S 300 Blue TEC HYBRID.[19]

These data very clearly point out again the causes of this planetary environmental pollution taking place right in front of our eyes – sorry, noses:

A product *stinks*. Or, let us be a bit milder, does not smell good.

In this condition, it won't sell.

So, the manufacturer plasters a lovely, attractive smell over the top of the bad smell.

And so, it sells and makes the customer sick.

This is as true for the automobile industry as it is for the industry of body care and household cleaners, let alone the industry of perfumes (that are supposed to cover "bad body odor" so that a potential sexual partner will want you).

Cindy is, therefore, developing into a sniffing junkie, whether she wants it or not. She also breathes the perfumes of her colleagues.

Since an attractive male colleague works not too far away on his computer, she rushes off to powder her nose in the bathroom. After all, you never know what fate will deliver. Cupid could strike quite unexpectedly. She smiles at the colleague as she hurries past him. He reacts with definite interest.

In the toilet, she is once again bombarded with perfumes, as we already know. Here she meets a cocktail of detergents and fragrances, but the penetrating smell of the detergents is no longer perceived – it is superseded by the stronger chemicals of the perfumes. Other ladies also regularly spray their perfumes in here.

Cindy draws out a small perfume bottle of her own and sprays certain regions. The name of the perfume is promising: "Aphrodite's Secret." Perhaps the Greek goddess will stand by her side when she walks past her colleague again.

She also applies an antiperspirant, a roll-on deodorant, because when she gets excited, she sweats a little. Cindy has no idea how this substance causes the skin's surface to change: the glands can narrow, or even become clogged.

In an investigation of forty roll-on deodorants from supermarkets, drugstores, and pharmacies, *Öko-Test* was only able to recommend *a single* roll-on deodorant without reservation. Thirty-nine were at least problematic, and some were crammed with poisons. Even highly toxic aluminum is found in some roll-on deodorants, which can also be found in some pots and pans. Some of the harmful substances found in *Öko-*

Test in deodorants/antiperspirants can lead to tissue inflammation, damage to the liver and acne.[20]

Back to Cindy:

Well, so be it! After all, if it is about love, you have to make sacrifices.

Consider the case of the truly obsessed woman, who may even know about these dangers about perfume, roll-ons, etc. but does not care because she is on the "warpath," intent on ensnaring a mate.

However, in the case of a more sensible woman, as represented here by our Cindy, she knows nothing about the harm she is doing to her body. She has no guilty conscience about her "fragrant" life. She considers that these are the usual and necessary precursors to attracting her man.

She re-applies her scented lipstick. Then she sashays proudly and, apparently, unapproachably back to her workstation, giving that impression, as someone once described it, of always "pulling" that sends men crazy.

And so, the day goes by. Unfortunately, the fish does not bite.

What she does not know is that this handsome colleague, who is in tip-top physical condition and enjoying good health, is also food-conscious, does a lot of sport in the open air, says no to drugs and excessive alcohol consumption, does not smoke, and avoids using perfume.

He has unconscious instincts that work well, and which tell him, as Cindy dances past:

"She smells wrong. This does not suit you. Steer clear!"

The Evening Poisons

After work, Cindy rushes straight to her fitness center. However, she does not know that perfumes have long been used in almost all studios. Once again, she sniffs poisons, though she thinks she is just getting her body into shape.

The physical training regime she favors forces the gym clients to inhale deeply and firmly. Cindy gets a mild migraine. She is prepared for it – after all, she has done this for two years now. She hurries into the changing room, where she takes a pill from her pocket and places it in her mouth. She then rushes back into the gym.

Finished with her work-out, she takes a shower with scented soap.

Now dressed again in perfume-laundered clothes, she decides to go and buy something. The department store is also perfumed. Accompanied by subliminal, beguiling music, the perfumes motivate customers to open their wallets.

Cindy only wants to buy something for her nephew, whom she adores and whom she will visit today. He has been coughing for a few days. She feels she should spoil him. She does not know that even some children's toys (as well as kindergartens) are already perfumed and contaminated. The air in some German kindergartens, according to an investigation carried out by the company *Lino Diagnostic* in Nuremberg, is already excessively contaminated by pollutants – even *Der Spiegel* has written a report about it.[21]

Her nephew may even develop asthma with his sniffing of further poisons and perfumes at home. The fact that this child comes to "enjoy" perfume is ensured by his mother and probably 99% of all mothers. She washed his bedding last night, of course using softener – the product containing the most fragrances in the entire category of washing aids.

His aunt, our lady Cindy, is no different. For a full nine hours, while she is in bed and asleep, she draws molecules of the fabric softener perfumes into her lungs and thence into her bloodstream and every cell of the body. Her bedroom windows are shut. She loves to keep warm. As usual, it will be with great effort that she gets out of her bed in the morning, still feeling tired, despite the nine hours of sleep.

One day, we will tell her that for a restful, healthy sleep, the most important element is fresh, clean oxygen. But let her sleep now, despite all her mistakes. It is not her fault. Thousands of psychs have programmed her environment so that, like millions of other people, she stumbles through life irresolute.

Perfumes Everywhere

Hopefully, by now, you get the message. Today, we encounter perfumes in all possible (and some seemingly impossible) places. In the nursing homes, in the waiting rooms of doctors, in fitness centers and airports, perfume poisons are pushed at us. The air is suspect in hotels and youth hostels, clubs (discos), kindergartens, health resorts, hospitals, schools and swimming pools (in addition to dangerous chlorine chemicals). We come across perfumes in taxis and public toilets. We find further perfumes on papers, books, magazines and plastic products.

It is a little-known fact that there are around 4,000 chemicals included under "perfume." 95% of these chemicals are extracted from petroleum – the oil industry plays a dubious role in this. Hand-in-hand with chemistry, it marches in a highly questionable direction.

The most amazing information, as I mentioned at the beginning of this chapter, is that *more than 80% of these chemicals have never been tested, as far as toxic effects on the human organism are concerned!*[22]

Eighty percent! Do you understand the enormity of this statement? The perfume industry is not regulated by any single government in the world. It is not obliged to provide information on the actual ingredients of its "odors."

In other words, we have merely described the tip of the iceberg here.

Our information is incomplete. It can only be incomplete because thousands of tests do not exist. They cannot exist because the substances, the chemicals that are contained in perfumes, are not even declared and are not known. At the same time, the perfume particles, the poison particles, migrate to the most remote areas on planet Earth. Right now, we are systematically contaminating our planet. For all our apparent abundance of worldly goods, we labor hard to make our organisms, our human bodies, sicker, and sicker.

The perfume and chemical industries are nothing but greedy crooks!

Can we stop this development?

How?

The First Possible Solutions

At the end of this book, when all the facts are on the table, I will present various solutions that will allow you to act immediately and effectively.

The enormously good news is this:

You can always do something about it.

It is my creed that one should not burden a person with bad news only.

I do not want you, the valued reader, in this case, to join the ranks of the catastrophe industry, which paints everything black until one is almost stifled and apathetic because of all the insoluble problems. That would create an effect of "world-weariness" to the extent that one finally throws up one's hands and does nothing at all.

So, let me introduce here a first solution, which at least allows you personally to avoid this attack on your health.

Checklist: A Fragrance-Free Home

This checklist is fully detailed in the last chapter of this book. You can work through it point by point. It will allow you immediately to move into action. If you take heed of this advice, daily, unwanted self-poisoning can be brought to an end, or at least banished from your personal space.

Although the points on this checklist are easy to read, from my own experience, I warn you that they will not be so easy for everyone to carry out 100%.

First, you will be shocked at all the places you find fragrances – and you may not perhaps always like to part with things that you have bought with your hard-earned money.

Your health, however, will thank you, and it is not impossible that some of the ailments from which you have suffered will disappear magically over time.

As mentioned above, please find this checklist in the final chapter of this book.

Rehabilitation of Your Olfactory Instinct

Living a perfume-free life for a few weeks and months will automatically re-set your instincts. After that, you will no longer consider perfumes as pleasant smells but will correctly perceive most of them as rather unpleasant. If this effect does not occur, you can be sure that there are still sources in your environment that emit chemical toxins into the air, such as:

- Indoor poisons (like formaldehyde, etc. from carpets or furniture)
- Toxic substances (plasticizers) that are emitted by cheaply manufactured plastic products

These are, likewise, generally dangerous poison sources, like perfumes. Therefore, they must be identified and handled.

In the future, when you are shopping, perform a quality control check on any product you wish to buy: **smell it!**

Your instinct will tell you whether the product is a danger to your health or not.

Likewise, with products bought online. What's the first thing you should do upon delivery? **Open and smell it!** If you consider it to be dangerous, immediately return it to the sender and let him know why!

A few years ago, I returned five air purgers I had ordered online. The reason: they all emitted more toxins than they could "clean" from the air.

Of course, you can do much more. Many methods work well of extracting poisons already present in your body. I shall write about these methods later – please be patient with me.

Once we know that chemically produced perfumes are extremely dangerous to your health, it is now essential to ask why. In the next chapter, let us have a look the way that perfumes affect our human organisms and what they trigger in terms of sex.

Let us firmly grasp this particular stinging nettle.

*Optimist: A person who does not
see things to be so tragic as they are.*

KARL VALENTIN
German comedian and writer (1882–1948)

CHAPTER 5

The Insidious Sexual Seducer: Perfumes

WE NOW KNOW that perfume surrounds us in every nook and cranny and that in perfume, there are found numerous poisons which can lead to all kinds of diseases. This revelation means, of course, on the other side of the coin, that with this book in your hands, some diseases might also be relatively easily cured – perhaps, even an existing condition from which you may be suffering.

We still do not know exactly how perfumes work. We do not know the exact mechanics of how they persuade us. HOW do perfumes fool us? There are certainly a lot of well-kept secrets to be uncovered. When we do discover how we are deceived, we will have invaluable knowledge that will protect us from this manipulation.

So, how does the olfactory system work?

(*Olfactory*: of or having to do with the sense of smell.)

There is a consensus among scientists that the sense of smell is even older than the optical (sight) or acoustic (hearing) sense. From an evolutionary point of view, we probably had a very good sense of smell before eyes and ears developed. The sense of smell is the most basic of all senses.

What exactly happens when we "smell" something? Well, in the upper part of the nasal cavity lie the so-called *olfactory mucosa*, which is about five cm² in size. It has about 350 olfactory cells, also called receptors. Each olfactory cell is programmed for a specific scent or groups of fragrances. Different receptors can be stimulated at the same time so that we can perceive *combinations* of fragrances.

When we inhale, molecules of substances present in the air are transported over the air to these receptors. The receptors, in turn, report what they sense directly to the brain via nerve cells. So, we immediately and without delay, know what something smells like. The message is direct without detours. Certain odors alert us to dangers, a warning which allows us to back off. Pleasant odors make us want to approach something.

It is a remarkable fact that there is no relay station between the olfactory mucosa and the brain.

Therefore, the message to the brain takes place in a fraction of a second – nothing is "filtered" or "thought through" again. And therein lies the rub. We do not *get* to "think" about odors.

They hit us directly. We judge them immediately. I shall speak of the enormous consequences of this in a moment. It is more than explosive.

Let's start with a few hard facts. The palate can only distinguish a few tastes, five in number: sweet, sour, bitter, salty and umami (the latter having been detected rather recently by Japanese researchers; the word "umami" represents a meaty, savory deliciousness, and as a taste, it hints at the plant and animal proteins). In contrast, there are more than 500,000 fragrances, not all of which can be differentiated by the average human nose. The possibilities for differentiation are nevertheless almost infinite.

Firstly, something smells good or bad. The smell is pleasant, or something stinks. An object can smell aromatic and fragrant or nose-wrinkling and disgusting. Then, more specifically, something smells of (say) roses, tulips, carnations, curry, or camphor. More and more distinctions are thus made.

If we want to describe specific odor perceptions, we immediately make comparisons. We can distinguish between numerous plants and flowers if we train our nose just a little bit. We can also distinguish between different species of animals and even between people, all of whom have a distinctive odor.

Woods and trees have a specific smell but, above all, flowers offer a vast range and great richness of odor. It is a kingdom of olfactory perception, enthusiastically spoken about in novels and poetry.

There are a few highly qualified people today whose sense of smell is so well developed that they can:

- perceive odors over long distances
- clearly distinguish between thousands of different odors.

Smell-geniuses! Some people even have an excellent odor memory (which can also be trained, by the way).

Literature is full of examples, as of men who recall the erotic smell of a lover, for instance, and sigh deeply over the memory.

About body smells, many pages could be written. A pleasant odor attracts; a bad one repels. Have you ever smelled a baby, paying attention to the smell? Incredible, isn't it? Have you, on the other hand, consciously smelled an old, sick person? What a difference. One signals the beginning of life; the other the approaching of death.

Back to biochemistry and the incredible abilities of our bodies: When it comes to food intake, aromas reach the throat and the nose, then progress to the receptors of the olfactory mucosa.

So far, around 10,000 flavors have been discovered, of which about 2,500 have been artificially produced. But do we only perceive through the nose as far as odors are concerned? Only a few people know that even sperm can perceive a smell, as recent research has found. The nose is not the only thing with this gift. It's not just the world of the nasal mucous membrane!

There is, no doubt, a connection between the sense of smell and the god Eros, which brings us to the following subject.

Perfumes and Sexual Attraction

Advertising, as well as literature, is full of examples which point out the connection between a person's odor and physical and sexual attraction. No one seized upon this link faster than the perfume industry, and of course, this knowledge was instantly abused by it.

Eau-de-Hongrie, "Hungary water," was the name of a perfume that was mixed around 1370. According to the legend, a monk created this concoction for the aging Queen Elizabeth of Hungary. It consisted of rosemary and lavender oil. This monk, a kind of Hungarian Rasputin, assured her that her beauty would be preserved "eternally." It was said that "Promptly, the seventy-two-year-old queen seduced the king of Poland."[1]

Of course, here we are dealing only with a romantic legend. Many charlatans in the Middle Ages, not just in modern times, fooled naive women (and men) with pills, perfumes and miraculous cures. Many comedies are based on such stories.

Literature is further well-stocked with novels and narratives in which erotic smell and perfumes play a role. The Irish writer James Joyce, for example, describes in his work *Ulysses,* a young girl who perfumes herself with musk scents. When her suitor appears, the following happens, according to Joyce:

> *"Yes and then he asked me would I say yes my mountain flower and first I put my arms around his neck and pulled him down to me so that he could feel my breasts all perfume yes and his heart was going like mad, and yes I said yes, I will Yes."[2]*

(The lack of punctuation was one of the techniques that made Joyce famous.)

There are also countless commercials which indicate that the right perfume is responsible for attracting the other sex. Like moths to the flame, women or men are supposed to flock to a person if he or she smells a certain, erotic way.

One could fill volumes with examples. Even the names given to perfumes are a giveaway. Here are some famous perfume names:

Dans la Nuit (at night), Amour Amour, Scandal, My Sin, Femme (Lady), Fille d'Eve (Daughter of Eve), Ocean of Love, Daughter of the King of China, Joy, Harem, Fancy Love, J'Adore, 212 Sexy, Desire, Eros, and so on and so on.

Using every means possible, the equation Perfume = Erotic has been hammered into the heads of men and women. It is more than suggested that if one "perfumes" "correctly," one has a better chance with men or women and will be more sexually attractive.

Even the flasks in which perfumes are stored (usually called flacons) send a clear message. A bottle was initially been made of polished glass, shaped with a narrow neck and a round belly. But, not infrequently, perfume flacons are also shaped in such a way that the message (sex and eroticism) cannot be misunderstood. Some perfume companies even try to reproduce feminine forms with their flasks.

Others choose the color black for their flacons, while others present both flasks and perfumes in front of a bright red background. Black and red are the colors of love and sex. Some perfume bottles are shaped like famous sex symbols. Everything that can directly or indirectly be associated with eroticism is used. Flacons have been given the form of men in fancy dress, and women's bodies draped in enchanting clothes. They have been decorated with representations of nudes, lingerie, and erotic scenes.

The packaging of the bottles is also essential. Boxes bearing a painted heart, for example, hinted at moving in the "right" direction. And, to warm up the women's market, the fashion industry hires sex-symbols for advertising. Seductive film and television stars, those who possess the greatest sex appeal, have often sold their names for a wad of cash.

Catherine Deneuve, Michael Jackson, Omar Sharif, Frank Sinatra, Joan Collins, and others have doubtless earned small fortunes. Nightclub kings, designers, stars and starlets from the music industry as well as supermodels have also been marvelously marketed.

A massive advertising effort has been and is being made whenever a new perfume is released. The most expensive market researches are done, trends are observed, surveys initiated. Everything, everything must be correct, especially the name, which is sometimes sought after for years – and for which one hires the most expensive advertising agencies and top-notch copywriters.

Even famous painters have made themselves available in the service of the perfume industry. Salvador Dali is just one prominent example. Simple advertising designers were replaced by famous artists who could swing their brush in their unique way.

Only the most famous and expensive photographers were sought when it was necessary to launch a new perfume.

The focus was almost always sex, sex, sex. Once again, we cross paths with the psych. Psychologists were regularly consulted to capture an erotic atmosphere. The serpent as a seduction symbol, identified by C. G. Jung as a symbol of the sexual act, served as an eye-catching visual on posters, advertisement, and commercials.

The effort was, and is, immense – but as long as a perfume is successful, it pays off, and millions are made.

From the earliest times, when perfumes first became profitable (and were still produced from natural ingredients), perfumers tried to figure out what were the most erotic types of fragrance. The plant and animal worlds were sharply observed, with a precision that was the envy of even the most famous artists.

To capture the "right" flower scents, it was necessary to pick the flowers when the buds had just emerged in their full glory as blossoms.

The right kind of *flower chronometers* was developed. These were precise timers that show which flower blossoms open at what hour. At that exact time, they had to be harvested immediately by the flower pickers, so that the highest quality perfume could be obtained.

Leaves, stems, flowers, fruits, seeds, woods, barks, mosses, herbs, grasses, needles, twigs, roots, and fruit peels were carefully examined. Again, and again, the perfumers were searching for the unbeatable aphrodisiac, which could stimulate and increase the desire for love.

Certain animals produced a musky substance from glands near their genitals, and this substance undeniably affected humans, too. Musk was already used in ancient times as an aphrodisiac. So, people hunted animals for their glands to add to perfume.

One such species, the musk deer, was hunted in Tibet and China. The musky scent was found in a pouch near the sex glands of the male musk-deer. The animal was continually feeding on aromatic herbs. In the rutting season, the male exuded such a strong odor that it could be detected by a female over many kilometers. Thus, the sinfully expensive musk was purchased for large sums of money and transported thousands of miles, often through secret paths and circuitous routes to avoid theft.

The substance called *civet* is similarly famous and infamous. The North African civet cat releases a strong-smelling substance from a gland near its sexual parts, which can likewise be mixed with perfume to make it last longer. Allegedly, the civet gives off an Oriental scent.

Castoreum was also highly sought after. This substance was discovered in a skin-pouch near the anus of the beaver. Castoreum was a favorite as an ingredient in men's perfumes, to produce leathery or tobacco fragrances.

Today, synthetic musk is produced industrially. Synthetic perfumes prevailed from about 1850 onwards. Even the rarest odor formulae were now synthetically produced by chemists. In chemistry, the word *synthesis* refers to the construction of a substance from simpler, different elements. Every possible flowering fragrance and all possible animal odors were deciphered and artificially produced, namely with chemicals.

Some small notes on biochemistry: iron, calcium, and the like are minerals, yes. The body needs minerals, yes but it requires them in biochemical (living) form, as they occur in (living) plants and fruits.

Dead minerals (metals, stones, etc.) cannot usually be used by the body. They can sometimes be used, but only with extreme difficulty. Otherwise, we could happily eat mineral-rich stones, earth, and sand or even coke – not from bottles, but as a derivative of coal. If this were possible, it would provide a solution for all famine. Alas, it isn't possible!

Vanilla, jasmine, violet, and especially musky smells, nature's great secrets, have all been discovered. Chemists have consequently embarked on frenetic missions to find more erotic products. Every perfume company nowadays has thousands of fragrance recipes at its fingertips. Every perfume recipe is treated like pure gold and kept strictly under wraps. The god of Eros almost always plays a prominent role.

But one must ask in all naiveté, what is the truth about the story of the connection between perfume and sex?

Secrets of Animal and Human Olfactory

When scientists first tried to trace smells, in addition to the floral kingdom, they targeted the animal world.

It was already known that not only the big cats, but also domestic cats mark their territory using scent. A cat who rubs against someone's leg is leaving its mark with its fragrance glands. Scent marks also serve as a "language" between animals. Some animal species communicate using scents!

Honeybees share some information using smells, as do skunks and ants. Ants mark their paths with formic acid. An animal fragrance also serves as a form of sexual luring. "The pig digging for truffles does this in the hope of finding sexual partners. Truffles are an aphrodisiac, because, like axillary sweat of man, they contain the sex hormone *androstanol*."[3]

Well, that's what our Cindy from Chapter Four should have known. Perhaps things would have worked out better with her armpit sweat instead of the deodorant. Probably the handsome colleague from the office would have reacted differently because then his instinct would have absorbed the real, true biodata. This would perhaps have irresistibly attracted him because the optics were undoubtedly right. She was an attractive girl – but, sadly, her roll-on deodorant killed off her *androstanol*, preventing what could have potentially been a great relationship.

"[Different] butterfly species lure their partners to them over many kilometers with fragrances."[4] The survival urges of the breed, the need for reproduction, seems to be the goal of these natural perfumes.

Other female animals ready to conceive sprinkle urine, which presumably contains distinctive fragrances, to signal to the males that they can be successfully mounted.

The fragrance glands of some animal species are particularly well-developed during the mating season – those of the beaver, for example, or the musk-deer. The beaver spray the already mentioned *castoreum* around to lure female beavers and to interest them sexually. Fragrances in the animal kingdom serve to mark out territories, attract sexual partners or, in some cases, deter enemies. The spray secreted by the skunk would be an example of this. It is used to instill fear in their would-be predators.

Human beings also have their fragrances (so-called *pheromones*) to lure sexual partners. In this case, they are called *sex pheromones*. A pheromone is a messenger for information-transfer between individuals within one's kind. Certain substances are thus delivered to trigger a specific type of

reaction. Science has uncovered the nature of the sex pheromones used for sexual stimulation.

What scientists have not yet confirmed, but what I (and others) dare to speculate, is that a woman radiates these aphrodisiac pheromones only or especially at the time of ovulation
(potential conception).

Allow me to digress. We need to develop a small, technical device that detects and reports these fragrances. This
would give us a contraceptive method with no side effects.
For couples wishing to have a baby, we could find the right
day for their contribution to the preservation of the human
race. Our instincts have seriously become shriveled. If we
had cherished them over the centuries and cultivated them
as did the animal world, we would not have to use small
technical devices but could rely on our sense of smell for
contraception.

In humans, in addition to the sweat glands, the glands of the
armpits are especially important. Also important are specific
enzymes (which are basically *converters*) that change odor-
precursor-molecules into the final odors.

Sweat, however, can also be unpleasant – a circumstance that
perfumes seek to remedy – but we can nevertheless at this
moment state that certain natural fragrances, both in the animal kingdom and among human beings, serve very well for
sexual stimulation.

The worst is yet to come, but let's hold off a little longer. Let us first examine the controversial topic of partner selection in the case of man.

The "Right" Partner

Again, to Cindy from Chapter Four: Why did she cast an eye on that colleague? There were many other possibilities in her workplace. Could she have smelled him? We remember that the nice gentleman was perfume-free. His body odor was natural.

While more and more seemingly rational criteria are now being applied to the finding of the right partner, it must nevertheless be noted that there are also genetic constants which play a role as to whether one or another person is found to be congenial and finally is chosen.

The famous butterflies in the belly that you may feel when you fall in love are at least partly dependent on genes. Women primarily, scientists have determined, make sexual decisions according to the dictates of genetics. Why?

"Every female creature is looking for optimal genetic make-up."[5] That is, a woman instinctively rejects men whose hereditary history is not optimal for her offspring. It is believed that women can smell chemical messengers in the man's sweat – on a subconscious, instinctive level.

Interestingly, women seem to be particularly suited to men (and vice versa) who have a gene pool that is entirely different from their genes. In the case of genes, too much similarity is unfavorable. Diseases can be better repelled by combining different genes. According to this theory, the female is looking preferentially for partners who, as mentioned, represent a completely different gene pool.

Mother Nature thus seems to have evolved the human female body to respond to male body odor in a way which is survival-friendly for the offspring. In reproduction, therefore, the *difference* is essential. For example, the Max Planck Society discovered that parasites could be more easily repelled if genetic resistance systems changed. Immune systems in men which differ significantly from the immune systems of women are preferred. One could speak of an immune-genetic supplementary program for the offspring.

Men are also partly exposed to the reaction of specific genes. Researchers have found that even sperm may absorb lily-of-the-valley scents, and the prostate is susceptible to violet scents.[6] Lily-of-the-valley (among other fragrances) causes the sperm to move in a particular direction. That is, within the approximately 30,000 active genes that we own, a part is programmed to respond to fragrances.

Also, in both sexes, the skin and the gastrointestinal tract can absorb odors – this is currently being energetically researched. Fragrance molecules also act via the respiratory system and thus on the lungs, and not just through the nose but through the mucosa. The lungs, in turn, deliver messages directly into the blood.

The fact is that every person has a very individual, unique body odor, which is influenced by one's genes. Therefore, family members often smell the same or similar.

On the other hand, smell sensations also depend on education and culture. A scent that is perceived by a person in Asia as pleasant may be described by another person in Europe as unpleasant. Even individual experiences play a role in fragrances, as Professor Hans Hatt discovered at the Ruhr University in Bochum.[7] Someone could, therefore, hate or love a particular perfume because of their life experiences.

This fact is of real importance. Our instinctive, innate smell system is designed to protect us. It promotes our survival. It should help us make the right decisions – and this leads us to a highly interesting insight.

Liars and Cheaters: Perfumes

While our olfactory system provides us with valuable information, whether it is through the nose, the sperm, the prostate, the skin, the lungs, the blood or the genes, this system can also be compromised.

By nature, we can differentiate good from bad and instinctively make correct decisions. A person who smells bad, or who does not fit in with us, a situation that literally "stinks," will soon be banished from our environment.

Perfumes, however, cause us to make mistakes, simply because they supply false information to our instinctive systems of evaluation. Perfumes make us "nose-blind."

Since odors evoke affection or dislike, we may end up giving our affections to the wrong (perfumed) person. We are also no longer aware of the dangers of the environment when a place has been sprayed with perfumes. The whole smell-safety system is thus extinguished when we operate with artificial odors. Fragrances fool us.

Quite apart from the fact that we absorb toxins in vast amounts through perfumes, whereby our health is slowly but surely destroyed, also our instincts are continually being manipulated.

And so, regarding perfumes, we see ourselves faced with the most unbelievable scam mechanism one can imagine. In this particular way, our instincts and our natural responses are eliminated. We are almost hypnotized. One of our most essential perception channels is blocked. Once again, we are fed with wrong information and so are bound to make wrong decisions!

With perfumes, we are constantly being steered in the wrong direction. Each of us is left stumbling through the sensory world like a doubtful traveler who has lost his bearings. One could classify the weak human in this situation as a kind of puppet or automaton, which can be arbitrarily pushed in one direction or the other. This "robot" is controlled by others through the seductive signals of perfume. One is no longer self-determined.

This alone would be dangerous enough, but further consequences are much more dramatic.

Suffering aside,
Diseases as an index are quite helpful.

OLIVER HASENCAMP
German writer (1921–1987)

CHAPTER 6

What Nobody is Talking About: Misdiagnoses, Invented Diseases, and Allergies

OVERALL, THE SCIENCE of academic medicine today spreads a sense of optimism. They give the impression that they know what diseases are and how we must deal with them.

It is true that *surgery* has made incredible progress. Just a few days ago, a neighbor, a doctor by profession, explained to me how he had sewn a torn arm back on. A few days before that, he told me how he had made the fingers of a shattered hand functional again and explained why he does not use silicone, but rather body-tissue for breast implants, because it is a much safer option. A broken leg nowadays is far from being a life-threatening problem, and so on.

All of this is to be respected!

But if you look at diseases like cancer, strokes, headaches, nausea, rheumatism, or various allergies (or apparent allergies), one must realize that our scientific medicine is still fumbling entirely in the dark. Might this have to do with the fact that our medicine is strongly controlled by professional pharmacists?

I think so. But this is not the theme of this book, except to say that simple solutions for diseases are not popular among the pharmaceutical industry. Billions can only be earned with medicines, not with curative methods that do not require medication.

An "allergy" is often merely the result of poisoning. Dr. John H. Tilden goes even further. The title of his book says it all: *Toxemia Explained: The True Interpretation of the Cause of Disease*[1]

However, if an allergy (or illness), is psychological, neither the doctor (with his scientific background and pharma medication) nor the naturopath (with herbs and alternative therapies) can help you. Nor can the psych with his psychotropic drugs.

Let us focus on the solutions and not the problems. If a doctor says "allergy" or "virus" or "flu," alarm bells should ring loud and clear.

Prepare for a trip into real life:

The Ignorance of Doctors about the Danger of Perfume and Respirable Volatile Chemicals

On a late autumn day in the 1980s, my then-wife and I planned a weekend visit to my parents in the countryside near Munich.

The week beforehand had passed with pleasantly warm temperatures, but toward the end, it grew noticeably colder. We were in for a cozy weekend in their warm house. On Friday evening, when I phoned my father, the world was okay. But on Saturday morning, when we arrived, his wife, my stepmother, lay sick in bed.

My father also did not look very fresh and lively. Worried, we entered the house to look for my stepmother. On stepping indoors, we were immediately hit with an offensive odor: the fumes of lacquer paints.

In response to my questions, my father explained that, because of the sunny weather earlier that week, he had spontaneously decided to paint all the window-frames before the onset of winter. A lightbulb went on in my head. A whole chandelier of lights switched on for me!

We went to my stepmother's bedroom. There was the same ghastly smell, owing to vapors from the paint. My stepmother was in misery.

"Why don't you open the windows?" I asked, mildly.

My father replied that, because of the cold temperatures, he had, of course, closed them, before the paint was barely dry.

Well, you will have guessed it already. My diagnosis was simple and expressed in good Bavarian:

"This toxic sauna here would knock out a bull-elephant, let alone my step-mum!"

I was amazed that my father was still standing. I could not have lasted in that atmosphere more than an hour, irrespective of which room of the house I was in.

I immediately opened all the windows and doors without bothering about how cold it was outside. Then I explained to the two of them what they had done wrong – but that they did not have to worry. In a couple of hours, after a few hundred breaths of fresh air, things would visibly improve for both, especially my stepmother.

This measure and the diagnosis seemed too easy for them, so I agreed that they should also consult with their scientifically trained family physician for their reassurance.

Said and done.

Upon his arrival, more than half of the paint-vapors were already gone, but it was undoubtedly still smelling strong.

However, the "learned" diagnosis of the doctor, who looked young enough to be fresh from medical school, was as follows:

"Well, there is another flu virus going around, which you must have caught. I will prescribe you some medication for the symptoms."

After I had explained the situation to him and the quality of the air as we had found it, I asked:

"Don't you think these paint-fumes could make one feel unwell?"

"No, no. Viruses cause this. They're just making their way around," was the response.

I quickly realized that a discussion was futile. The boy had his clearly defined, stubborn routine for his diagnoses: symptoms, viruses, flu, drugs. Finished!

Our doctors seem to be studied experts on drugs but have never learned about the body being a carbon-oxygen machine with a duration label on it, and that this duration label gets drastically shortened when you put wrong or even poisoned food (carbon) or poisoned water, or poisoned air (oxygen) into it. His only excuse might be that there are no medicine universities in the world that teach nutrition and biochemistry. So, rightfully, we must point the finger to the educational system of our doctors.

So much for the competence of many doctors regarding diseases caused by poisoned air. Let us get to the core of this. The word "allergy" is often used in similar ways by doctors. It is just as skillfully pulled out of the hat as "viruses" and "flu." I might become a very popular country doctor in the Bavarian backwoods without having studied for twelve semesters, as follows:

In the case of all headaches (or blocked airways, fever, head-ache and so on) you say this: "Well, there's another virus going around."

"What virus?"

"Very hard to say. But I'm prescribing these new pills for you. They'll cover the whole spectrum."

In the case of all aches and pains below the neck, the formula would be as follows:

"Hmm, this looks like an allergy. Take these five drugs for three months. If it's still there after that, then we'll do an allergy test".

In severe cases, best use the following (said with high authority):

"You must go *straight* to Professor Vitzliputzli in the district hospital."

The patient is then transported at high speed to the hospital, with blue lights flashing. This looks like a good thing to do, as in a movie.

And then occasionally, depending on the "fashion" of the moment:

"Ah. You are predisposed to the recently discovered Tohubohu Disorder."

What can we say to that? Well, I think there is a subject that could be given the title of "Artificial Diseases."

It sounds even better to speak of "mental disorders," or, for example, ADHD (Attention Deficit Hyperactivity Disorder). Also, more frightening still, "depression" is a popular buzz-word in the current vocabulary.

Note that it is claimed that these "disorders" can be treated very quickly – and irresponsibly – by many doctors. In parallel to the invention of these "disorders," the pharmaceutical industry also happens to have the "right" psychotropic drugs to hand to "cure" them. These are marketed through the network of general medical practitioners. Compared to the money made by medical pharmaceuticals, the profits from illegal drug networks of the largest Colombian cartels look like peanuts.

At one point, a doctor in the Arnstadt region of Thuringia said the following when I discussed this subject with him: "Yes, I know, these are not real diseases. But what should I do? A youngster comes to me and expects that I am going to write a sick note and prescribe him such-and-such a psych drug. If I do not, he goes from doctor to doctor until he has found one from whom he gets what he wants."

Has this doctor ever looked up the word "responsibility"?

The reason for this incidental dissertation is that I once lost two good apprentices from my employment because of psycho-pharmacy. They were not dismissed by me. After a few weeks on psycho-pharmaceutical drugs, they were no longer able to work. They became social-welfare cases. Now, they cost decent, hard-working German taxpayers a few thousand Euros per month.

My God, what a huge market this psycho-drug market is! And who in the world, especially at a young age, does not feel "depressed," (i.e., in a bad mood) from time to time?

Depressions in the good old days

At a certain point, I wondered: how were similar problems solved in earlier times when there were no psych drugs? Hmm!

I remember my first "depression." I had a broken heart. My friend Walter happened to be in the same boat at the time.

What did we do? We consoled each other over a few beers, followed by some glasses of liqueur. Then we cursed and vented. And at about two o'clock in the morning, we staggered home, laughing and singing.

That was on a Saturday evening. On Sunday, we had to play in a football match. Action was demanded. Again, on Monday morning, we had to be back at work. Once more, action was required. There was no time to ponder. We did not have time for "depression."

If everyone who ever suffered from lovesickness went to a prescription-writing, money-grabbing doctor, and filled themselves up with psychotropic drugs, we would soon have 100% of our population on such drugs. Then, goodnight world. Who would be able to work?

Repeat: Allergies

But back to our main thread. Although it is widely unknown how allergies come about, there are long-standing therapies that can be used to relieve allergies effectively. So, expect some *good* news.

But first, we really should try to find out what allergies are. Let us ask ourselves in all innocence:

"What is an *allergy*?"

The word itself comes from Ancient Greek, where *allergia* means *foreign reaction; allos* means *different, strange, peculiar.* It is a defense reaction of the immune system to something perceived as foreign and dangerous to the body – a *peculiar* defense reaction, however. Sneezing would be the best example.

The immune system responds to certain environmental substances (allergens), with inflammation of the area which encounters that substance, for example. Symptoms may occur only seasonally or all year round.

An allergy can manifest as hay fever, show up in swellings and skin problems, in diarrhea, and more. A person may be allergic to animal hairs, pollen, plants and trees, house-dust-mites, foods, and so on. Oh, and of course, *perfumes* can also trigger allergic reactions – which brings us back to our theme.

Nothing but Facts

Perfumes ("fragrances," "perfume," and "aromas," etc.) can lead to allergies, so it is known. Let's take a closer look at that:

Chemically produced perfumes lead to diseases. This happens more slowly in one person, faster in another person. Nobody, however, becomes healthier by inhaling perfume. On the contrary, everyone then has to deal with more or less weakened health.

But let me quote what scientists today state without any ifs and buts:

- Allergies are now a global health problem.[2]
- Numerous scientists see the cause of increasing allergies in the continuous increase of perfumes in cosmetics and household products.[3]
- Perfumes are now regarded among the five "top allergens" by scientists in North America and Europe.[4]
- People who are repeatedly or regularly exposed to perfumes are at risk of developing allergic symptoms at a later stage in life.[5]

Although the full truth is perhaps even more dramatic, at least these four facts above cannot be shaken. The investigations are too precise and too careful to dismiss as trivial, worthless, or inconsiderable.

Details

Let's look at the details. On average, a perfume contains more than ten unknown (intentionally secret) chemical combinations consisting of literally thousands of chemical components, which are not listed on the label. Some of these substances not only trigger allergies but are also responsible for many other ailments.

66% of the substances kept secret have *never* been checked for their suitability for use by humans, i.e., for possible damage to health. Even the chemical substances that *can* be found on the labels have not been thoroughly investigated. Factually, 19% of known and declared substances were never tested for their health risks.[6] In other words, the consumer cannot possibly make a rational decision about a "good" perfume, even if he takes the trouble to put his glasses on his nose to decipher the fine print. Every time he wears perfume and then goes to bed with bed sheets washed with perfumed laundry detergent, he's playing Russian roulette.

Perfume in the bed linen and perfume under the armpit of the partner and various other body areas, as well as freshly washed hair with perfumed shampoo, means that sex can be perilous.

After all, one breathes deeply in and out during the act. Within a few seconds, the chemical perfume particles reach the brain cells. Ever had a headache during sex? Or a migraine afterward?

Some of us have an intuitive sense that "something is wrong" with a partner. But is it wrong with *them*, or their smell?

Perfume can even influence vital decisions.[7] I know a man who instinctively parted from his wife for no apparent reason. The hidden bane was the perfume she wore!

Perhaps it is worth investigating the proportion of separations which occur due to perfume. I dare say perfume could play a part in quite a few separations and divorces, on an instinctive level. The mind, of course, is looking for a rational explanation and will conjure up the wildest justifications that the abandoned partner cannot understand. Unfortunately, detailed investigations of such possibilities do not exist at the time being. And such an investigation would be very difficult in the first place.

Once more: Allergies

Allergies can arise even from the most expensive and classy perfume products. Whether it's a product by Giorgio Armani or whether it is promoted by Halle Berry or Jennifer Lopez, perfumes contain toxins that can make us sick and bring about allergies.

These hidden, secret chemicals are also found in the most popular perfume brands, radiant with the celebrity and status of idols like Britney Spears or Coco Chanel. The corresponding poisons can still be absorbed or inhaled through the skin and lungs. The effect is the same – we come into contact with toxins whenever we operate with perfumes.

Recognized allergic effects include headache, a tightening of the chest, diarrhea, and vomiting in children, asthma, dermatitis, and irritation of the mucous membranes.[8] A pretty, colorful palette, don't you think?

The Trick of All Tricks: Greenwashing

I do not rule out that perfume manufacturers have long been aware of the problem. Some try to cover it up because it could hurt their finances.

Scientific cited research above has never been disproven, simply because it cannot be disproven. So, different perfume manufacturers try to toss sand into the customer's eyes. How?

By labeling perfumes like this: "pure fragrance," "organic fragrance," or "natural fragrance."

None of these expressions can be legally criticized – that is to say, in many countries the manufacturer can designate anything as "organic" or "natural," without being called before a court because these terms are not protected by law.

Our advertising psych can, therefore, continue with his old game of abusing traditional, honorable words as a sick joke. Just as the "German Democratic Republic" was formerly neither *democratic* nor a *republic*, so are today's perfumes neither "organic" nor "natural."

Thus, the *psych* uses good words badly, to spread his poisons. He poisons the words themselves to be able to sell his health-damaging products. Since most perfumes, even if they are now chemical, artificial and toxic, were sometimes originally obtained from Nature, one can, in one way or another, refer to "herbal ingredients" (plant extracts), to herbal extracts, or "natural" constituents. What does *not* come from Nature is not mentioned.

The unwitting customer trying to avoid synthetic chemicals is sold by these misleading words. Even perfume products that boast labels stating "perfume-free" or "natural" or "organic" or "gentle to man and environment" or "eco" still sometimes contain fragrances.

A Wolf in Sheep's Clothing: Ecover

Allow me to make a small comment on the British brand Ecover: When I moved to the UK in 2008 and searched for a washing-powder as one of my first purchases, I came across a health food shop, where, I assumed, everything would be free of perfumes. I found washing powder by the brand Ecover. My thought was, this is "eco" and it is in a health food store, so it must be good. I did not have time to study the list of ingredients, so I bought it.

What did I discover at home a few days after my first use of it? Synthetic, chemical lemon smell. "ECOver – Powered by Nature" was on the pack. But when I did bother to read the small printed list of ingredients, sure enough, "fragrance" was among it. I have not yet experienced a more insidious wolf in sheep's clothing. This led me to contact the PR department of Ecover. What did they tell me when I brought my complaint to them?

"Well, none would buy it otherwise. The customer demands a bit of scent."

Where's the morality in that?

The lady on the phone seemed to be very knowledgeable and certainly, must have known something about the potentially toxic effects of manufactured perfume chemicals on the organs of the body. But instead of enlightening customers and offering them non-toxic products, they promoted their poison products under a sneaky cover that pretended to be part of a clean, safe environment! How unfair is that?[9]

There are other brands like Persil, where all you are told is:

"… with spring fragrance."

It is, in a way, more honest. In the legal sense too, nothing can be done about this: the perfume maker is (still) within legitimate grounds. So, it only helps to clarify that it contains toxins under the umbrella of "fragrance."

And Once Again: Allergies

In the Research Institute for Fragrance Materials (RIFM), thousands of fragrance ingredients are listed, of which *at least 100* are known as allergens. The RIFM (New Jersey, USA) is considered to be *the* international scientific authority about the health-damaging effects of fragrances. Over 112,000 studies have already been carried out within the framework of this research institute.

The range of allergens in the RIFM is continually being expanded as the industry adds new chemicals to new perfumes, meaning new perfumes are invented and concocted using all kinds of ingredients. Several fragrance chemicals have even been classified as carcinogenic and harmful to the immune and nervous system. As always, new allergens emerge.

But stop! Can one not identify allergens through a doctor? What a pretty illusion. If an affected person tries to consult an expert – a dermatologist, for example – to be tested for allergens, he or she is usually disappointed.

Why? Tests exist for only a small number of all the possible allergens. Only twenty-six substances can be so identified today, no more. In most cases, the visit to the allergy 'expert' is therefore not crowned with success.[10] Many patients who complain of specific problems (headache, dizziness, nausea, etc.) do not even know *that* this is an allergic reaction.

We have not even talked about the fact that even a positive allergy test – for example, a skin reaction – does not always mean that *all* allergens were detected. *Several* substances can be responsible for an allergy. A perfume (or a cleansing agent) can consist of several hundred individual elements. Also, a person is usually surrounded by *numerous* perfumes, cosmetics, and cleaners. So, you can see immediately that you are a hopeless optimist if you believe that, by testing, all the triggers for an allergy will come to light.

At the same time, the use of perfumes is continuously increasing, as poisonous fragrance spans the entire planet like a fine haze of smell. In the meantime, ingenious inventors are coming up with alarm clocks that can wake up the sleeper in the morning with "coffee" smells and devices which, when playing computer games or in the home cinema, emit certain fragrances that are supposed to fit the action.[11]

Yes, there are twenty-six known fragrances which have been shown to cause allergic reactions, which must be categorized by law if they exceed a specific quantity. But this is not nearly enough. There is an abundance of tests and standards missing.

Regarding irritation of the respiratory tracts, there are far more tests than those that deal with irritation of the skin. But, as Dr. Wolfgang Straff from the German Environment Agency asks:

"What happens when you have finally found an allergen substance within a product – but exactly which one it is, the manufacturer of this product cannot determine?"[12]

So, it is not surprising that, in certain professions, allergies have long since continued to rise.

Professions at Risk

According to the official list of the German Professional Association, the following professional groups are particularly at risk:

- Bakers
- Hairdressers
- Masseurs
- Caregivers

In these professions, a person often comes into contact with dusty food chemicals, flavors, and cosmetics. It is not surprising that more than 5,000 cases of "Baker's asthma" and a further 5,000 cases of allergic skin diseases are reported annually to the Trade Association by professional associations.[13]

I repeat: EVERY year!

In addition to these dangerous professions that have been officially confirmed, I would like to add the following:

- Perfume Shops Sales Personnel
- Flight personnel – the captain as well as attendants (air quality in airplanes needs great improvement – and it is not because of the dry air, as is stupidly claimed and justified by airlines!)
- Any cleaning services (mainly laundries)
- Restroom attendants
- Hotel staff
- and many more

How much more proof is necessary before the legislature prescribes effective, stringent requirements or even better, entirely forbids chemically produced fragrances?

The situation is terrible. But my creed consists, as I have said, of not only spreading bad news. Much more important is *good* news.

As far as the subject of perfume energies is concerned, there is a simple, excellent message for those affected.

But please be patient. Let me give you a few more facts.

How Allergies Come About

Following the arguments put forward by Dr. Mauch, let us first look and ask ourselves how allergies can develop in the first place.

Well, perfume poisons enter the body, especially from deodorants, which are sprayed, powdered or rolled under the armpit. Under the armpits, there are many pores, including lymphatic nodes, which (unfortunately) work to keep these toxins evenly distributed over the lymph drainage system that covers the entire organism like a net.

Substances within the deodorants then react with minerals that are naturally present in the body, to form harmful salts. These salts subsequently accumulate in all possible body parts and lead to chronic inflammation and the first "allergic" reactions.

Inflammation, as much as is known today, is found more frequently in acidic environments. The body forms defense mechanisms, which leads to redness, itching, and pustules, for example.

Long-lived perfume poisons and other environmental poisons are constantly being added to the body. Additional new toxins, which may be contained in detergents, for example, or in other cosmetics or wherever, enter and react with the old, stored toxins. New chemical reactions now take place between the new and the old toxins.

The body goes crazy. It no longer knows how to master all these poisons and reactions. As a result, sudden, violent, "allergic" reactions arise such as the runny nose, conjunctivitis, or asthma. The equation is, therefore:

Poison plus poison = allergy.

Thanks to the researcher and alternative medical doctor Walter Mauch, attention has been drawn precisely to this way of producing allergies.[14]

Let us repeat it because it is so important!

According to Dr. Mauch, who has examined hundreds of allergy patients and returned them to health, allergies are due to poisoning. These are caused primarily by deodorants sprayed under the armpits because from here they spread particularly fast through the organism.

Suddenly, one day, the new poisons react with the old poisons. The possible number of reactions is unlimited due to the abundance of toxins that exist. Theoretically, one could perform hundreds of thousands of tests – and make the topic inconceivably complicated.

However, if you keep the matter simple, you immediately realize that many different reactions can take place between various poisons, to which the immune system reacts desperately and in a hectic manner because it wants to protect the organism.

Allergies indicate that something is wrong in the body. The immune system defends itself. It raises a warning flag, which cannot be overlooked. The human body informs its owner:

"Something is up. Attention! Something is wrong right now. Do something quickly!"

Allergies are, in any event, due to *poisoning*, and it must be added that even inferior-quality food can contribute to this poisoning because our foods have long been "flavored," i.e., poisoned with artificial aromas, as we know by now.

If one has understood the basic principle of where an allergy comes from, the riddles which many doctors are still struggling to solve to this day dissolve suddenly into nothing. Theoretically, if one understands the phenomenon, one does not have to lose oneself in a thousand nomenclatures and make the topic infinitely complicated.

Every truth is simple.

The Perfume Danger

Let us summarize the facts in a simplified but precise way:

Chemically produced perfume is a toxin for every organism.

Perfume reduces the quality of the air we breathe.

These chemical substances do not belong in the air or the water. For millions of years, they were not there.

Our bodies are used to good, clean air. It is necessary that air remains of good quality. Any contamination weakens our health to the precise extent that the poison has entered the air. The atmosphere may tolerate a little poison, but your health and your immune system are weakened by these perfume poisons.

The more and more frequently you are exposed to such poisons, the more destructive it is for your health and your immune system.

We are dealing with a very simple equation. If you do not believe it, think of a very simple test. What if you were to go to your garage, close the doors and windows and turn on the engine of your car? The chemical substances from the exhaust pipe would gradually poison the air in the garage. The poison would rapidly make you sick and sicker. If you did not remove yourself in time, you would die. This equation is so simple.

The above example is very quick poisoning through the respiratory tract. It is almost painless because you become tired and lose consciousness before death.

Perfume poisoning, on the other hand, is much slower than car exhausts. But it still works. Depending upon the quantity of perfume and which particular ingredients are used, it acts faster or slower. The result, however, is always a weakening of your immune and other bodily systems. The result is almost always a disease. However, it is many times more painful than our thought experiment about the dangerous "test" with the exhaust gases.

You can expect:

- Sneezing (this is probably the best and most pleasant reaction. The body defends itself and tries to expel the particles as quickly as possible from the body)
- Headaches
- Migraine
- Respiratory irritations and infections
- Anything from a runny nose to 'flu-like symptoms
- Allergies and even cancer (after twenty, thirty or forty years of daily perfume intake), as some experts have noted.

A more comprehensive list of possible diseases caused by perfume poisoning can be found in the book by Dr. Walter Mauch already mentioned, *Die Bombe unter der Achselhöhle* ("The Armpit Bomb").

So, these are the effects of perfumes as far as your physical health is concerned. Also, there are psychological effects. Here is a small list:

- Your mental awareness "shifts down a few gears," so to speak.
- Your alertness and attention span are reduced.

- Negative emotions take possession of you.
- Expect irritation and nervousness.

This happens especially when you know nothing about perfume. One feels a danger instinctively, yet it remains unknown, which can even lead to anger. One is looking for a cause or a culprit, but since one does not know about the danger of perfume, inevitably one aims at wrong causes or the wrong culprit. Unnecessary disputes with a partner or friend are often the result.

Sometimes a feeling of wanting to "run away" from a place or a person may arise. I do not rule out that this can sometimes end in serious tragedies. "Running away" from a partner (I am speaking of divorce) can be the result because one can no longer correctly sense him or her.

Now, back to the previously mentioned good news:

Remedy for Perfume Allergies

As long as an allergy to fragrances is not due to a psychological cause (and many times that is not the case), then you can get rid of the allergy by running the **PERFUME CLEANSING** Checklist which you will find in Chapter Thirteen of this book.

All these actions require what could be called the "mature and intelligent patient," who *wants* to become active himself or herself. Such people do not allow themselves to be swallowed up by a passive, pill-popping mentality which implies that just by consuming the right droplet or pill, all will be fine.

This is one of the most prominent lies of our time. It requires self-initiative and perseverance to return to health – but only the stubborn ones win the battles, something that Napoleon was aware of.

Even though perfumes involve many toxins, it is vital to keep in mind that there is also good news. There is a solution to every problem. There is a fascinating amount of know-how that leads to health. But first, you must recognize how substances act upon you, and with what result.

However, we are now standing with one foot already in the next chapter. So, turn the page, please.

A healthy lifestyle is uncomfortable to begin with
but comfortable in the end.
With an unhealthy lifestyle, it is the other way around.

GERD UHLENBRUCK
German immunologist and aphorist (1929–)

CHAPTER 7

What the Smell of Perfume Does Not Reveal or: The Truth About Hormone Disorders

THE DANGER WITH perfumes is that they fog our senses and give us a false sense of health and hygiene when the exact opposite is the case. They contain poisons. Perfumes can cause disease, as we have seen in the subject of "allergy." However, the full extent to which perfume poisons can affect our organism is unknown.

The Hidden Facts

Increasingly, today, "irritations" of the hormonal balance of animals and humans are occurring around our planet.

In his eye-catching film "Chemiefalle" (Chemistry Trap), aired on March 11, 2007, by the broadcaster Phönix, the author Claus Hanischdörfer pursued some inexplicable phenomena of the animal world. Even in natural paradises like the Alps or in the Lake of Thun, all is no longer as it should be.

Together with Professor Helmut Segner, a hormonal specialist who teaches at the University of Bern, he found:

Almost half of all whitefish [a species of salmon-like fish] caught ... had significant malformations of the genitals. Somehow, highly toxic chemicals had entered into what was considered a 'clean' reservoir of drinking water, which supplies around 400,000 people. The testes of the fish in this lake were altered in some way; there were also above-average numbers of hermaphroditic[1] fish and many deformed sexual organs.[1]

Let us look at a second example. In Florida, scientists found that in a specific lake there were hardly any alligators to be found, although they should have thrived there. The reason? The few eggs that were found and examined were contaminated with chemicals, specifically with hormone-modifying substances. Also, male animals had become more female.

A third example. At the North Pole, polar bears and seals were contaminated with chemicals and pesticides. Polar bears were increasingly born as hermaphrodites.[1]

And so, we could go on and on, but we believe you have understood the message long ago. The fact that hormone-active substances are now threatening the survival of the animal world

---

1 hermaphroditic: having both male and female sexual organs

(and also the people) is currently without a doubt. Pesticides in almost all waters are the official miscreants.

Even tiny amounts of hormone-active chemicals can have a negative impact on sexual development. Many animal tests have also confirmed this suspicion. Fish in the waters affected by chemical waste lose their fertility. But is it only the pesticides?

Hormone-modifying chemicals are found today in packaging, in computers, in shoes, in the car, in children's toys and, of course – you have already guessed it – in perfumes. The increasing infertility of men in some areas of Europe is, in my opinion, directly linked to the "perfume trap."

For this, I spare you the list of my sources. Just Google it and enter a few keywords. There are plenty of horror reports. The tests were carried out over many years on people who were, on average, thirty years old.

Currently, infertility is increasing rapidly. One should compare this trend with the sales statistics of the perfume industry, or with the use of perfumes in these groups of men. I am sure that you can identify correlating trends here. The more perfume, the more sterility.

Of course, at the time being, this is an opinion. Specific research needs to be done on this. But the data at hand strongly hint that perfume is the cause for this rising infertility.

The chemical industry is ultimately responsible, but the perfume industry is a branch of the chemical industry. The approximately 100,000 existing chemicals which the chemical industry has now put out into the world have never been checked for the harm they cause.

Scientists estimate that about two-thirds of these chemicals are harmful to health. We are talking about more than 66,000 poisons.

Let us repeat: 66,000!

In this context, I will restrict myself to perfume chemicals only. Perfumes are used close to our bodies and therefore, are among the most dangerous. It is also clear that chemicals that have a devastating effect on the sex hormones have been discovered in perfumes. In my opinion, one can hardly imagine what one day will be found if one were to carry out *comprehensive* tests. The following is already known by professionals:

Only for the expert
and those who want to know exactly

The following substances, which can have an adverse effect on sex hormones, have been found in perfumes:

octinoxates, oxybenzones, benzophenones 1 and 2, diethyl phthalates, butylated hydroxytoluene, galaxolides, tonalites, musketoons, benzyl salicylates, benzyl benzoates, Lilial [2]

A beautiful register of sins! These perfume chemicals disturb hormonal balance. They can disrupt the production of hormones, their release, and their movement within the organism, as the scientists Gray and Rudel have proved.

Some chemicals can also imitate hormones, simulating their activity in the body. They then emit hormone-like signals at the wrong time and to the wrong tissues. As a result, overweight and thyroid problems can arise, as well as issues with certain glands.[3] Hormone problems, in turn, can lead to cancer, the horror of our time, especially prostate and breast cancer. And, yes, the corresponding (hormone) poisons can also exert an influence on the fetus. Even birth defects can be the outcome, just because of "simple" cosmetics we use[4] or the daily synthetic fragrances to which those expectant mothers are subjected.

You think you're in a bad horror movie, but unfortunately, it's a reality.

Am I, perhaps, exaggerating?

The Protest of the Industry, or Caution: Trap

Of course, the chemical industry vehemently disputes such accusations. It loudly demands long-term tests, which allows certain products to continue to be sold in the meantime. These long-term tests would, of course, according to the chemical industry, have to be carried out by the chemical industry itself, at its own expense.

Should we leave these tests to the chemical industry?

What happens when the wolf accused of eating sheep is appointed his own judge? Right! He will, of course, be freed from all charges. He will claim never to have eaten a sheep. He will put on a black, brilliant, good-looking judge's robe and make a false judgment, as he is the accused. It would cost him millions, even billions of dollars, if it turned out that he regularly tears sheep apart and devours their flesh. The chemical industry, as its own judge is not feasible.

What about all the professors and doctors as well as the legions of experts and scientists? Oh, this is again the hottest of all topics. I'm afraid I must rob you of a pretty illusion.

The truth and nothing but the truth is that by now many professors, doctors and "experts" with their various respected titles have long been on the payroll of the chemical industry. The fact is, in today's society, with the right fee, one can get many professors to agree to any statement. It is simply a question of how much. A professor usually costs more than a doctor.

This has been well documented for the pharmaceutical industry by the authors Kurt Langbein, Hans-Peter Martin, and Hans Weiss.[5]

In other words, the difference between "pure research" (tests falling into the field of research with no idea of "more preferable" or "less preferable" results) and "industry research" (tests hoping to find results which will please industry) is increasingly blurred at the moment. This is because industry can offer large research grants. And a professor who is on the payroll of the chemists will hardly contradict his employer or sponsor, nor will he wish to discredit him with "bad" results. He would immediately be branded as a traitor and would have to pick up his hat and leave.

This moral pressure or bribery of many scientists has long since been well documented in many other areas, such as archaeology, history, even physics. This does not mean that there are not highly honorable scientists, but it does mean that the word "scientist" is not above reproach. The beautiful goddess "Science," whom we worship everywhere today, is not infallible.

He who puts enough gold on the table can affect things in his favor. So, unfortunately, the truism remains true that he who pays the piper calls the tune.

The Neutral Researcher

Fortunately, there are still fully independent, highly respectable scientists (including chemists) and doctors whose real effort is to help and heal. And some poisons, such as phthalates, are increasingly being researched by such, and their adverse effects are indeed being linked to perfume use and abuse.[6]

Of course, one can also point a finger of blame at the neutral researcher for not always judging objectively. And, unfortunately, there are subtle methods of getting rid of him, for example by torpedoing any possibility of his publishing his findings.

But there is still a single, incorruptible judge – reality.

Bearing this in mind, it is quite remarkable that a physician will achieve surprising successes in healing his patients if he would only:

1. stop perfume poisoning, and
2. apply methods and techniques aimed at detoxification.

Dr. Walter Mauch, for example, considers the connection between perfume toxins and hormone disorders as 100% proven. He has personally observed hundreds of patients in his practice, and finally found:

Cosmetics, especially deodorants, enter the hormonal organs through the lymphatics, coming from the armpits, and disrupt the hormonal balance of both men and women and block their hormonal metabolism. Hormone disorders and osteoporosis are separate diseases that have the same cause – poisoning by chemicals – and therefore arise at the same time.[7]

Am I of the opinion that all existing hormone disorders are due to poisoning? Certainly not. But there should be some thought about the upswing in the hormone industry in recent decades.

For a while, the discovery of hormones was celebrated as the *ne plus ultra* of all health insights. Besides, hormone therapies have been and are increasingly being praised as a fountain of youth and as the method to beat old age and aging.

Hormones, hormones, hormones! Even the idea of the andropause, the male counterpart to the female menopause, is seeming increasingly attractive and is currently being promoted more and more in advertising. Men's andropause has long been a bubbling business and income source for particular doctors. It would be worth examining this phenomenon whereby the challenges and problems of one sex are apparently being repackaged and sold to another. In a free society, an individual should have some choice about what gender roles they play and to what extent, but instead, various industries seem determined to manufacture and steer these roles *en masse*, not for our greater freedom or benefit but only for their profit. Much "feminization" of the male world and, vice versa, the tendency to try to transform women into "better men" rather than competent women might be examined in this context.

There are, quite possibly, very different reasons for everything of this kind that has so far been sold to us. The simple fact that "hormone disorders" could be a poisoning process is, in any case, usually overlooked.

Theoretically, this opens the door to an entirely new field of research. We should look more closely at *poisoning* than has been done so far.

According to Dr. John H. Tilden, a twentieth-century member of the Natural Hygiene movement which started in the 19th Century in the US, all diseases begin with poisoning of one kind or another. In his book *Toxemia Explained* he describes the cause very extensively.[8]

I fully agree with him. This doctor, like no other, has reduced "diseases" and their appearance to an easily understandable, simple point. To restore health, he rarely prescribed drugs, but used fasting cures! He naturally made implacable enemies for himself out of the AMA (the American Medical Association) and the even more powerful pharmaceutical industry.

However, with my previous contention that all diseases are caused by poisoning, I must add the following caveat – there are also mental diseases, that is, caused by the mind or the soul.

Let us now go on with the text; we have only just begun to leaf through the book of sins of the perfume manufacturers. Let us now approach one of the most carefully guarded secrets of our day, which can radically alter our understanding even of history.

*Psychologists are people who understand
the soul as much as nothing.*

CHRISTIAN SCHYBOLL
German Author (1952–)

*Therefore, he did not hate anybody as fervently as
the psychiatrists, who thought they could dismiss
all his difficult behavior with a few foreign words.
(From The Man Without Qualities)*

ROBERT MUSIL
Austrian Writer, 1880–1942

CHAPTER 8

Perfumes, Psyche, and Psychoses

SEEMINGLY, *SEEMINGLY*, PERFUMES lift our self-awareness. We smell better and perhaps have a better chance with the other sex. That is what we believe in our great simplicity because that is what is advertised, so therefore it must be true!

In our *minds*, we feel more alive, fiercer, and more energetic when we spray ourselves with perfumes, while in truth we are saying goodbye, on the physical level, to vitality, energy, and fitness. We *seem* to be able to buy all possible emotional characteristics with perfumes: "freshness," "sexiness," and even "innocence."

The "innocence scent" is supposed to attract a specific type of man, apparently, while in reality, people are only fooling themselves – trying to cover the sun with a finger. More precisely and clearly, they have surrounded themselves with poisons. All these false promises now affect us in different places, not only in TV advertising. Magazines are also fragranced; sometimes, even, perfume strips are placed in them – perfume strips whose fragrance we take in without our consent, encouraging us to buy, buy, buy.

Such perfume strips are, fortunately, rare. But have you ever noticed that high-gloss magazines straight from the press sometimes smell of chemicals? No? Then, next time you go past a magazine shop, open one of these magazines in the middle pages and put your nose into it.

Please do not breathe too deeply. After that, you should exhale quickly and firmly. Brilliant colors need chemicals. The average customer has still not reacted to such magazines. They have not protested.

If this information is spread around, that alone should be enough. The health-conscious reader will begin to avoid printed magazines more and more. However, the advertising psychologist will whisper in the ear of the publishing companies of this world: "You only need a few fragrances – and your magazine will smell 'pleasant,' so long as you carefully avoid any hint of the poisons therein."

Other forms of paper are, increasingly, perfumed too, including letters and advertising mail. We live in an age of perfume.

As noted in previous chapters, these poisonous perfumes, no matter from what source they are emitted into the air, enter our lungs and brains via the respiratory tract. In the lung, they may lead to asthmatic complaints. Some experts say that about

75% of all asthmatics already have attacks triggered by perfumes.[1] In the US, this figure amounts to nine million people.

Let's stay with the psyche for a moment, which is also the subject of *emotion*. The insidious aspect of the perfumes is that some of the odors even penetrate the blood-brain barrier. This barrier obstructs typically all foreign substances from reaching the brain. However, some perfume molecules undoubtedly do reach into our brains, which gives them the potential to damage brain tissue.

This type of affliction is a type of neurotoxicity: *neuro* means *nerve*, *toxicity* means *poisonousness*. So, we must deal with *nerve poisoning*, which we create ourselves when we spray our bodies with certain perfumes.

A Revealing Comparison between Smoking and Perfuming

At this point, a comparison should be made between smokers and people who pour perfumes on themselves.

Why do I think that perfume could be more dangerous than smoking? In this comparison, we must also consider **asbestos**, a carcinogenic material that has been subjected to stringent legal requirements after the facts became known. During the production or demolition of asbestos panels (those grey, corrugated roof covers) dust is created whose particles are so tiny that they cannot be caught by the filter barriers in our nose when inhaling. So, they pass into the lungs. There, these particles bite like shards into the walls and cause lung cancer. Asbestos particles are small enough to be breathed in but large enough to be blocked by the lungs from traveling further into the body.

Tobacco particles, on the other hand, are smaller in proportion to asbestos but are still partially blocked by the lung with only some particles traveling into the bloodstream. When they do get into the body, they cause considerable health damage. This was denied by the tobacco industry for decades. They fought back and depicted these findings as unbelievable, unproven, and so forth. The evidence, however, is overwhelming. How many deaths through tobacco have taken place during this decade alone? How many millions of people have been robbed of how much quality of life and health? How many tobacco addicts are there still today? So, why is tobacco still not completely forbidden, or at the very least taxed much more heavily than anything else?

Furthermore, shouldn't the money derived from these tobacco taxes be used to pay to help alleviate tobacco-caused illness? In fact, why is the tobacco industry not already charged for these costs? Why do non-smokers and health-conscious people still have to pay for the health costs of these victims of the tobacco industry?

So, back to our beloved perfume. In principle, the cycle is similar to tobacco, but it is much more treacherous, insidious, and dangerous, just like a hidden bane:

Against the much smaller perfume particles, our body does not seem to have built an effective barrier. They are all small enough to pass through our lungs, into the bloodstream. From there, they penetrate the very depths of our cells and cause chaos in the truest sense of the word. Cells are biochemical power plants. But the biochemical elements of our bodies are not merely factories: they are alive, so to say without going too deep into biochemical expert know-how. So, they are part of a living dimension, part of the living universe, requiring life-friendly input.

Perfumes, on the other hand, belong to a category of materials which are more like asbestos, stone, metal, or the like: solid, hard, dead matter (especially the solid particles in aerosols). And so, they constitute part of the "unliving" universe where no real biological life exists.

To make the point again, in a simplified version:

Metallic iron, for example, dug out of the ground, is an entirely different substance from the biochemical form of iron that is found in fruit, vegetables, meat, and other foods and which, as a valuable mineral, fulfills essential functions in the body.

And, the metal-type particles, the unliving substances which are found in perfumes (chemically produced cocktails) have no business getting mixed up with the natural processes taking place within our biochemical, cellular

***power stations, our cells. They cause malfunctions up to
the point of the destruction of cells.***

Nerve Poisoning

Back to nerve poisoning.

Linalool, the most commonly occurring artificially produced
chemical poison in perfumes, is known to cause (among other
symptoms)[2]:

- breathing difficulty,
- lethargy and
- depression.

Lethargy can be equated with drowsiness, indifference, and
inactivity, including depression. Ha, *depression*! Here we are
again on the track of a very special secret, that we began earlier. Let us now enter a little deeper into this world of the
psyche. *Depression* is one of the most important issues of our
time. More and more people are suffering from depression.
This is Big Business, a real money-maker.

Psychiatry has numerous available pills which allegedly help
against depression. However, the unimaginable side effects
of these pills are mostly unknown. The alleged blessing of
the anti-depressants, however, is hammered into the heads of
human beings, again and again, every day, on every television channel. Apparently, these pills help against depression.

But there are also voices that claim something entirely different. Let us, therefore, illuminate the darkest, furthest angles to this argument.

What Is Not Said About Depression

Let us first clarify the word "depression." The dictionary teaches us that a depressed state has to do with sadness. Depression is described as an emotional state characterized by a feeling of hopelessness and sometimes the idea of personal inferiority.

Characteristically, there is furthermore a lack of energy as well as a difficulty in concentrating. Depression can also include destructive, negative thoughts, thoughts of death and suicide, fatigue, sleep disorders, anger and feelings of guilt, as well as the loss of appetite. It is indeed a colorful palette of symptoms!

The origin of the word is very interesting. It comes from the Latin word *deprimere*, which means literally "to push down, to depress." So, when you feel "depressed," you are seemingly pressed down by something or someone. However, no one has so far pointed out that this "something" could include the poisons in perfumes.

By the way, previously, *depression* was called *melancholia*, by, amongst others, Hippocrates, the famous Greek doctor. The word "depression" first appeared in the seventeenth century, but it only became popular in the twentieth and twenty-first centuries.

Today, depression is a lucrative business for psychiatrists and pill dispensers. The medical profession is very willing to prescribe medication if it promises to do something about depression. Of course, the psychiatrist has not refrained from inventing other "chic" expressions that are somewhat related to the word "depression."

He is a master of this, although thinking up a word for a type of conduct is by no means therapy, and not even necessarily a diagnosis. The psychiatrist today also likes to speak of "mood disorders" when he wants to interpret problems about emotional changes. This term is a new expression, which is likely to enhance his career as well because the psychiatrists now attach to everything the label "disorder," by which they always point to a "mental disorder."

They invent diseases on the fly! "Bipolar disorder" is an expression that is currently being spread and marketed by psychological and medical magazines, which points to the highest highs and deepest lows in mood. You could spend several semesters trying to beat through the undergrowth of all such fictitious words, which are invariably highly impressive and seemingly "scientific." However, let us concern ourselves specifically with "depression," which can be provoked by perfumes.

At the end of this chapter, I will once again present a small program that helps the person concerned to work himself or herself out of a depression in most cases. First, you must recognize how many words are buzzing around alluding to depression. There are hundreds of elevated, so-called "technical" terms. They are created by psychologists and psychiatrists and are formally labeled with intellectual-sounding names.

One thing you will not know is how to get rid of depression with a high success rate. In the typical situation, the patient receives prescribed some pills whose side effects are sometimes so strong that they can even provoke suicide. In the best-case scenario, the affected person may be sensible enough to stop taking such pills after a short time.

Allow me a little irony. If they do stop their medication, the sufferer finally and often joyfully returns to his normal "depression." He is grateful that he is *only* depressed. This is because only one condition is even more terrible than depression, and that is falling into the hands of a psychiatrist!

Psych drugs have components that affect emotions. How do we know these effects? A correct assessment would be to align them with alcohol, street drugs, and party drugs which have much the same result. This means that we are in the right category. Psych drugs are DRUGS. Let's not sugarcoat the pill – to coin a phrase!

I repeat: Some pills can either cause depression or worsen it. Then you need a pill against the pill. If this does not work, one needs a pill against the pill against the pill. And then, well, you can write the tragicomedy for yourself!

What You Need to Know as a Mother or, The Colorful Palette of Psychological Side Effects

If you follow the word "depression" along its destructive path, you can also see the many side effects of perfume drugs. If we then also consider the side effects of the psych drugs, we immediately recognize the vicious circle one may enter.

Some odors have psychoactive properties, which involuntarily puts them into the category of psychoactive drugs, not unlike the dangerous Prozac or Valium. There have been numerous physical as well as psychological side effects documented in the case of perfumes.

Headaches, especially migraines, watery eyes, anxiety, nausea, dyspnea (breathing discomfort), inability to concentrate, foggy feelings in the brain, dizziness, fatigue, a feeling of oppression on the chest, trembling and hyperactivity; all these symptoms can be encountered when you use perfumes.

Hyperactivity is a huge issue for children now. You could write your own non-fiction book about this. Children are particularly vulnerable when it comes to perfumes. A parent who is using perfumes can pollute the air that the child inhales.

In this way, a mother or a father can slowly but surely poison their child. These may contribute to or even lead to a loss of concentration, a learning disability, and the phenomenon of a fidgety child, as well as stunting the child's growth in extreme cases.[3]

This is no fiction. Researchers from all over the world are now reporting on this issue. The numerous investigations by those neutral experts who have not been enlisted by psychs, big pharma, chemical companies, or the perfume industry can no longer be ignored. Adverse effects have been documented in overwhelming numbers. In France, the USA, the UK, Denmark, Sweden, Germany, Austria, Japan – in all these countries, the mentally damaging effect of perfumes has been reported.

Chemists in toxicological institutes, authors of articles in specialized magazines which focus on specific health problems, and numerous expert books and researchers in independent universities speak clearly on the subject of damage from perfumes.

The *Toxicology Journal* and the *National Academy of Sciences* in the US have reported on the side effects of perfumes, as have the Danish National Environmental Research Institute, the municipal clinics in Dortmund, the University of Vienna, the Swiss Institute of Toxicology, the Swiss Federal Institute of Technology, and doctors in Augsburg. The number of sources is overwhelming. Not even a billion-dollar company can dismiss or deny all this evidence.

Everywhere, experts speak of "perfume toxins." There has long been suspicion of them playing a role in Parkinson's disease, Alzheimer's, and other neurological problems, i.e., nervous diseases. Questions upon questions suddenly arise, as far as chemical poisons in perfumes are concerned.

By psychiatrists, psychological problems have long been associated with "nervous conditions." I will not discuss this intellectually disputable position at this point. Theoretically, we could investigate numerous, further neurological diseases. A connection with perfume poisons cannot be ruled out. Let us quote only two statements to summarize the issue and to indicate the possible range of the debate.

In the fact sheet "Making Sense of Scents," it says:

> *"884 toxic substances were identified in a list ... of 2,983 chemicals used in the fragrance industry. Many of these substances are capable of causing cancer, birth defects, **central nervous system disorders**, breathing, and allergic reactions, and Multiple Chemical Sensitivities."*[4] [Bold print added by the author.]

Could you express it more clearly?

The fact sheet continues with:

> *"The chief reactions [to perfumes] we see are those that affect the nervous system - headaches, anxiety,*

depression. But anything can be affected, even diet and a personal intolerance for different foods. There are two significant ways in which cosmetics and their chemical constituents can affect the body. One is through direct contact. Inhalation is the other major route for molecules of an active substance to enter the bloodstream... There is a route from the nasal passage into the nervous system... It is the way, for instance, that inhaled cocaine affects the brain."[5]

This statement leaves nothing to be desired in terms of clarity. Again, and again, one finds references in the relevant literature to "mental" or "psychological" reactions regarding perfumes. This can have the following consequences: fatigue, a sense of confusion, headaches, loss of short-term memory, inability to concentrate, lethargy, anxiety, irritability, depression, unexplained mood-swings, and restlessness.

As stated before, it is a colorful palette then. And this is not to mention possible physical reactions, such as skin rashes, eczema, muscle, and joint pains, irregular heart rhythm or swollen lymph glands. It was the Candida Research and Information Foundation in the USA that compiled this alarming list.[6] The mental and psychological effects of perfumes are therefore well documented.

Perfumes can even partially stimulate psychoses, so experts tell us.[7]

But let us stop. We have heard enough *bad* news.

Let's take a deep breath and ask ourselves: What can we do about it?

Let us now introduce some *good* news to our creed and let us discuss how we can *effectively* address these ominous "depressions," which should be more understandable by now.

Let's turn the tables.

Understanding Depressions

First, it is essential to make a distinction. Depression can be triggered by circumstances that are associated with the psyche but also by certain *poisons*.

The first step is, therefore, to differentiate clearly. It would not be wrong to speak of "mental depression" on the one hand and of "body depression" on the other. These differentiating terms are used in this book as follows:

Mental Depression: a depression that has its effects on the mind and is caused by a real or imagined stress situation. They range from heavy stress such as oppression and sup-pression to lower levels of stress such as a crisis in love, grief due to loss such as the death of a close person, losing one's job and so forth. Such a situation can make the mind sick and subsequently, also the body.

Body Depression: a depression that has its causes in a deficient diet or poisoning. In the latter case, tiny quantities of poison accumulate so powerfully over time that the body can no longer cope with them (examples are drug residues, smog, perfume, chemical residues or additives in food, and so on). If you want to track down the cause of a disease, it is advisable *first* to check out possible body depressions.

The good news in this context is that I would say in my own experience that about 70% of depressions are body depressions. Their causes can be detected by simple means and can be quickly and effectively eliminated. Body depression can be made to disappear relatively quickly if the right actions are taken. Perhaps the percentage of body depression is even higher. Do you understand how exciting this discovery is? Most "depressions" can be cleared *much* more easily than we have hitherto believed.

Body Depression and the Remedy

Check and find potential poison sources in the following three areas and eliminate them.

BREATHING – DRINKING – EATING

On the topic of **BREATHING**, consult the two checklists in the final chapter of this book:

- **FRAGRANCE-FREE HOUSEHOLD**
- **FRAGRANCE DETOX**

On the topics of **DRINKING** and **EATING:**

If you find it difficult to locate poison sources, consult a nutritionist or a doctor who believes more in a healthy diet and fasting than in drugs. Or, roll up your sleeves and start in on the *Do-It-Yourself* method.

Here are some literary tips:

- Dr. John H. Tilden, *Toxemia Explained*

  Tilden, a member of the American Hygiene Movement, is the best literary reference I know for healthy eating and drinking, as well as for finding the sources of poisons.

  A side note: The Hygiene Movement in the USA originated at the beginning of the nineteenth century. Healthy, natural diet, and treatment methods such as fasting were the focus, making practitioners of Natural Hygiene the enemy of scientific medicine. At the beginning of the twentieth century, this movement was supported and revived by German physicians who had migrated to the USA, such as Professor Arnold Ehret, but it did not gain ground.

- A few decades later, Dr. Herbert M. Shelton tried to rebuild this movement. He renamed it *"Natural Hygiene,"* but he too had a hard time against the increasingly powerful pharma-funded AMA (American Medical Association).

Today, in the USA, the National Health Association (formerly known as The American Natural Hygiene Society) keeps the essence of this movement alive. See www.healthscience.org.

Also, these books are recommended:

- Guy Claude Burger, *Die Rohkosttherapie* ("The Raw Food Diet")
- Arnold Ehret, *The Cause and Cure of Human Illnesses*, as well as *The Mucusless Diet Healing System* and *Rational Fasting*
- other publications by Herbert Shelton
- Harvey & Marilyn Diamond, *Fit for Life* volumes I and II, which are a summary of Shelton's teaching

It would be presumptuous to attempt to reproduce the contents of these books here. I want to say that they can all help to get rid of depression finally.

Back to Body Depressions

The good news for the depressed is that in the case of a body depression, nothing is wrong with the individual concerned personally, nor with his or her ego – the "I."

Such a person is not insane or crazy. He or she is only suffering, very simply, from poisoning. A poisoned person is, apart from the toxin, completely normal, even if he or she reacts from time to time in such a way that some are quick to label him "neurotic" or even "psychotic." The analysis, the diagnosis, is, therefore, the first step in the process of depression. Never accept "depression" alone as a diagnosis.

Psychiatrists who eagerly prescribe psychotropic pills without divining a precise cause are becoming more and more discredited.

Mental Depressions, Tips

As I said, I believe that most depressions are "body depressions." Once the poisons have been discovered, they can be safely and efficiently reduced without problems. There are very many methods. They are all listed in the books mentioned above.

As to the remaining psychological reasons for depression, the following steps may help:

- One should deliberately and purposefully move away from or restrict contact with oppressive persons and "poisonous relationships" in one's life. Some authors write about people who only talk down to, depreciate, minimize, and criticize the person concerned, which can make a person feel sick and depressed.

- **Work (Action)**! Probably the worst thing you can do in a bad mood is to take sick leave. Usually, in such cases, the person concerned sits at home and begins to ponder. This is precisely what he should not do. This strengthens the depression.

  Action, on the other hand, even as much as sixteen hours a day, is beneficial. This means that one should pursue his regular work and also do overtime if it is available.

  If you must stay at home for a while, play sports with friends or do some gardening, or tidy up the garage, the attic or the cellar. It is also helpful to paint a picture, knit, engage in a craft, or do other creative work. There is always some activity available. Have you ever noticed that people who have a lot to do are usually mentally alert? Conversely, those people who have nothing to do are generally in a bad mood and less alert?

- **After work**. A person should, after work, focus his or her attention on something constructive and positive, such as a hobby which he or she has always wanted to pursue. Painting, writing, dancing, and gardening would be good examples.

- **A decision.** Help others wherever possible, thus drawing attention off oneself and onto other persons. In this way, one can find a purpose in life, which is also conducive to recovery.

- **Movement and physical exercise.** These are other methods to counteract depression effectively.

- **Do you have boxing gloves and a punchbag?** If not, then it is also possible with bare fists and an old teddy bear, unwanted by the children. Imagine the punchbag or teddy bear is the person that has caused you your trouble or the trouble itself. Hit it good and hard, targeting specific parts of the "body" until you feel sure they will not forget it.

A Gentle Way (in case of lovesickness)

- Enter a busy area, such as the pedestrian zone of a major city or a large event, a place where a lot of people are located. Stroll through the crowds or sit down at a place from where you have a good overview. Give yourself a cup of coffee. Look at all the pretty women, or all the handsome guys, depending on your preference. After a while, you will (hopefully) realize that there is, after all, plenty more fish in the sea. Realize that someone is also attainable for you.

- And then it's back to work. Action!

Short Conclusion

When all of this is done, it is likely that 90% of all your depression is under control.

Of course, there may be mental depression, which cannot necessarily be solved by these steps. But it is not the purpose of this book to present therapy for every kind of depression – that is a separate work.

Nevertheless, my remarks may serve to prompt us to look in a very different direction than pills. We should be more systematically alert for body depression. Body depression is very much the subject of this book. Hopefully, this way of thinking opens up completely new perspectives for those affected.

Statistics

The following facts and statistics should make one think: If psychiatrists and psychologists were to have the correct answers concerning mental disorders and depression, we would have less and less psychological conditions in our society. But statistics prove that our society has more and more mental issues.[8] These negative statistics are curving upwards at a frightening rate. So, what's wrong with psych drugs?

However, I do not believe that our population is becoming as crazy as such. We have recently experienced an explosion of new words and definitions of mental diseases. Psychiatry has been inventing them! New "disorders" are continually being forced upon the population, who can then be sold even more "magnificent" pills with their often incredibly harmful side effects.

In my view, it is not a matter of mental illness (although some diseases can unquestionably affect the psyche) but, as already indicated, it is very often a case of being given erroneous diagnoses. In my view, many or even most of these cases are caused by poisoning. The perfume industry, which must be regarded as part of the chemical industry, is, to a very large degree, responsible for this poisoning.

But that is not the only point.

The side effects of perfumes are even more than already stated.

That is in the next chapter.

We belong to a civilization that knows how to produce death industrially ...

CURT MARTI
Swiss writer (1921–)

Death goes two steps behind you. Take advantage of the lead and live.

WERNER MITSCH
German aphorist (1936–)

CHAPTER 9

Perfumes and the Grim Reaper

THEORETICALLY, ONE SHOULD be much less afraid of death than we are generally made to believe in our society. (That does not mean that one should agree with a painful, slow, and premature death from the effects of medical interventions such as chemotherapy.)

Those who have just studied the previous pages will have realized that some of the listed diseases caused by perfumes can lead to death. The range of possible diseases that can be triggered by perfume poisons is far more colorful than one might initially believe.

Dr. Walter Mauch writes of a large number of diseases which can be traced back to perfume poisons. He mainly points the finger at dangerous deodorants applied under the armpits. Here is a small selection of the possible perfume-caused diseases which Mauch and other authors have systematically compiled.

Be assured; this is only a *small* selection:

- Lead poisoning
- Breast cancer
- Bowel diseases
- Birth defects
- Skin cancer
- Bone softening/osteomalacia
- Bone loss/osteoporosis
- Cancer (other types)
- Multiple sclerosis
- Renal disease
- Brain damage
- Thyroid diseases

The path of the perfume to every cell in the body

The process, according to Dr. Mauch, is always the same or at least very similar:

Because of their minute size, particles of perfumes can reach unimpeded into any cell of the body, not only by inhalation but also, as already described, by simple skin contact.

If deodorants are sprayed under the armpits, where pores are wide open, poisons can enter the lymphatic system very quickly. The lymphatic system permeates the entire body. It is responsible for the body's enemies being repelled. It is part of the immune system. Below, two illustrations:

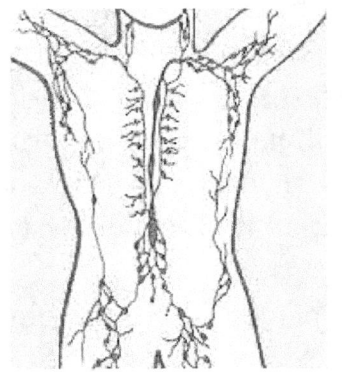

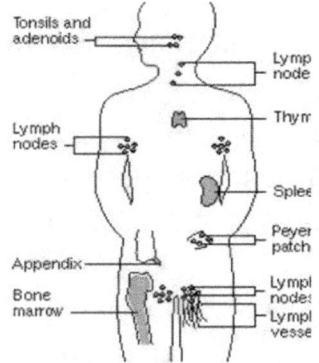

Lymphatic vessels   *Lymphoid organs*

Lymphae means *clear water* in Latin. It is an aqueous, light yellow liquid which forms an intermediary between tissue fluid and blood plasma.

Within the lymphatic system, about two liters of lymph fluid is transported per day. We could not live without this lymph system, because lymph and blood are closely related. Many things are transported by the lymph system, including fats ingested by the intestine, which are transferred into the circulation of blood.

The lymphatic system thus carries nutrients and waste materials, therefore helping to provide the body with valuable substances and clear it of "trash." Besides, it disposes of pathogens such as bacteria and foreign organisms. It has an invaluable double function.

Johann Kellerer

This lymphatic system is now being compromised by perfume poisons. Its fluid transports the perfume poisons to all possible parts of the body. The normal (positive) function (transport of nutrients and disposal of pathogens) is transformed into a detrimental (negative, harmful) service: Toxins are now systematically distributed to any location in the body system.

In each case, toxins may reach into places where the physical weaknesses of a person already lie. They may, for example, become lodged in overstrained shoulder joints, causing inflammation and even stiffness.

In the head, perfume poisons could migrate into the jaw, teeth, nose, forehead, eyes, and so on, causing all kinds of damage. If the ears are affected, loss of hearing, tinnitus and other damage can result, including earaches and a loss of balance.[1]

In the case of breast cancer, which is so often found today, one has to keep this in mind: lymphatic passages lead directly from the armpit to the breast glands. The poisons are not diverted. On the contrary, they form deposits in conjunction with certain body substances. The more perfume poisons are used, the larger these deposits can become. Finally, cancerous tumors may occur.[1]

A woman so afflicted, who feels she is in urgent need of a scientific doctor, will find perhaps that in determining the cause he uses a vague definition under the term "heredity" or will speak of a "genetic predisposition."

These "diagnoses" are no more helpful than "another virus is going around again," as mentioned previously. The highly qualified and well-meaning doctor is, proverbially, at his wits' end.

Physicians should, in my opinion, be more cautious in pointing out "genetic defects." A false assignment of cause prevents a further search for the real cause and precludes an opportunity for efficient healing.

How does it help if a person is told that they have cancer because their mother already had cancer? Such a statement does not open the door to healing, at least not today in 2019.

(I do not want to ignore the hope that modern medicine will finally build the perfect body genetically, but I guess it is still a few hundred years away.)

On the contrary, this approach promotes an apathetic attitude. Suffering or a physical problem is then deemed to be "in the family." This then might as well be labeled Karma, Kismet, an evil curse or the will of God, against which you cannot do anything anyhow. The fact that perhaps an incorrect diet could be the cause or even the same poisons to which both daughter and mother have been equally exposed is wholly overlooked.

"Overlook" – one could use the term apologetically at first. More precisely, however, it is more likely that these straight-forward healing methods and healthy lifestyles are not taught to our medical students. Why? Because there is no money to be earned from them!

So, where is our Health Department today? Ah, on holiday, in a resort on the North Sea, getting fresh air. And with him is a lady, with a perfume cloud ten meters in diameter. Forgive my sarcasm.

Back to Dr. Mauch: the lymphatic system can also transport perfume poisons into hands, feet, knees, hips, and so on. There, they are stored in pockets. This leads to inflammation and ultimately destroys the bone joints (arthritis). In the case of bone loss (osteoporosis), poisons are infiltrated into bones via the lymphatics, where they systematically decalcify them.

Heavy metals, lead and aluminum, play a decisive role – they are often the true villains.

Aluminum is found not only in perfumes but also in children's toys, tools, pots, and pans – our society is severely contaminated with this toxic metal. Whole books have now appeared on the subject. Aluminum is used in the cosmetics industry, especially in sun creams, in medicines for heartburn, and in two-thirds of all vaccines – we encounter aluminum everywhere today.

Aluminum is often found in cooking pans so that with every meal we import toxins into the body. Many waterworks add aluminum compounds to drinking water – this is supposedly necessary for its purification. The result? In your household drinking water, you may find aluminum residues. If so, it is a definite source of poison for your body.

Deodorants containing aluminum seem to be the main villain in this dark game, for aluminum modulates the immune system. And one final day, the immune system will finally collapse, as the organism protested in vain. At first, "only" allergies arise. But it builds up from there. While experimenting on animals, the systematic supply of aluminum even caused dementia.[2]

In any case, a person's health deteriorates rapidly. It goes systematically downhill, but there are other ways for the organism to protest. Dr. Mauch discovered that perfume poisons and chemical toxins could also lead to muscle and tendon infections.

As a result, the scientific physician may then speak with the weight of his experience as an "expert" to declare that the problem is due to, say, rheumatism. This seems to be a blanket term covering a wide range of symptoms. It is regarded as a highly practical part of our vocabulary.

Scientific medics do not fully understand what is going on with this ominous condition of rheumatism and will even admit this, to a degree. Nevertheless, the scientific medic eagerly prescribes pills for rheumatism to counteract the inflammation.

How much wiser it would be to:

1. Stop the drug supply and
2. Catapult the toxins out of the body that caused the problem in the first place.

Perfume poisons can thus damage bones and can also lead to disc discomfort or lumbago. They can also penetrate muscles and tendons.[3]

They can make the bowel sick. Lymph centers also exist in the intestinal wall. As a result, toxins will at first cause damage to the intestinal wall, and then further problems will arise.

The intestinal environment may change, possibly resulting in intestinal putrefaction or bacterial infections. Intestinal mycosis (including candida overgrowth) can also occur since the poisons weaken the whole organism. Mycosis, viruses, bacteria, parasites, and micro-organisms bloom when the immune system is no longer functioning optimally.

The conventional medics by now are looking at a host-body that is no longer able to strike back and defend itself. The intestine is particularly susceptible to disease. In the end, a nice mess is created. The doctor and the patient may subsequently kill off the bacteria and fungi, while the *foundation* upon which their proliferation has been based, healthy intestines, has long since ceased to exist.

The medical profession works hard on symptoms and illnesses which occur only after the second or even third tier of the toxic attack on the body. The real villain in the play is therefore not discovered. The basic starting point, the true cause, call it the first cause, remains hidden. The hidden villain is perfume as well as other toxins. The persons concerned unwittingly continue to spray themselves more and more with perfume poisons.

Our lymphatic system transports the toxins into the remotest corners of the body. Even organs such as the kidneys can be affected. The thyroids may be playing up and so on. One could enumerate a hundred diseases and each time come to the same conclusion. One would always discover the same Mephistopheles pulling strings behind the scenes – perfume!

Health Consequences: Premature Death

What is the result? **Illness and, most likely, premature death.**

I have already indicated it earlier. Perfume poisons can also cause cancer. We have already talked about breast cancer.

There are numerous types of cancer. That cancer can result from perfume, and toxin poisoning is now undisputed. The evidence is, indeed, overwhelming.

⋆⇥◉ ◉⇤⋆

Only for the expert
and those who want to know exactly

*"A few of the chemicals found in fragrances known to
cause cancer and birth defects: methylene chloride;
toluene; methyl ethyl ketones; methyl isobutyl ketone;
tert Butyl; sec Butyl; benzyl chloride"*[4]

⋆⇥◉ ◉⇤⋆

In other words, the chemicals mentioned above, which can often be found in perfumes, have been shown to cause cancer and birth defects.

The relationship between perfumes and cancer has been brought to the attention of various parties. Greenpeace has already raised its voice. Their experts, who are fortunately not on the payroll of the chemical industry, found that certain chemicals in perfumes may produce cancer.

> [They] *"may be capable of causing cancers or other adverse health effects ..."*[5]

Greenpeace noted that some plastics, children's pajamas, sports shoes, toys, and cellphones might also contain carcinogenic substances.

Newspapers have also reported that teenagers sometimes die through sniffing deodorants. A student put a bag over his head a few years ago and emptied most of a deodorant spray into the bag. Of course, propellants also played a role, which, by the way, can also cause a fire.

Bild headline:

> *"Mein Sohn hat sich mit Deo-Spray zu Tode geschnüffelt (My Son Sniffed Himself to Death with a Deodorant Spray)"*

And the text continues with:

> *"The boy with a gentle smile has gone without saying good-bye. "15-year-old high school student Fabian died alone in his bedroom. Unbelievably, the boy sniffed himself to death with a deodorant spray."*[6]

Nothing could revive him. Cardiopulmonary resuscitation, artificial respiration. Not even an emergency doctor who injected adrenaline into the boy's heart.

Other cases are also documented since numerous children have been seriously injured by deodorant sprays, which we have already established are sources of toxins. Much more insidious and, sadly, even more, important in terms of the numbers than such few but spectacular tragedies which hit the headlines is a general, creeping, deteriorating state of health.

Gradually, in the case of poisons, one's energy, one's physical force, is lost, which means that the organism can finally no longer resist.

Poisons overwhelm it.

Bear in mind that it is not just perfume-poisons that weaken the body. But even if other chemical poisons and drugs, as well as harmful medications, are considered, perfume poisons nevertheless often contribute a substantial complication to the fact that a person:

1. Sometimes falls ill with cancer.
2. May die from it.

Looking at it in the light of what we have uncovered, there is nothing less than our own and our children's health at stake, as well as the well-being of billions of people.

Why should a few perfume-manufacturers earn millions while poisoning half the world? The chemical industry should not be left unscathed and unaccountable.

At the very least, the industry should be prevented from continuously exposing the environment to further toxins without any controls.

Nobody can make me believe that these polluters do not know what they are doing. I do not want to know how many hidden vaults exist containing more detailed studies of the deadly dangers of chemically produced fragrances. If my presumption is correct, their behavior is entirely criminal.

Man becomes ill in an underhand way. Allow me once again to make an ironic statement.

If I were a terrorist and my mission was to eradicate the health and productivity of a particular country within (say) thirty years, I would do it with perfume. And the sting in the tail? Most likely, I would escape any punishment.

Neither the Minister of Health nor the Minister of the Environment is doing anything against these abuses.

But the subject of politics leads us to the interesting question of what the legal situation is.

Could we not – theoretically – sue the perfume industry?

And how do the watchdogs of the system, the ones who have real responsibility, react to our concerns?

I'll talk about that in just a moment.

The future has many names.
For the weak, it is unobtainable.
For the fearful, it is unknown.
For the brave, it is opportunity.

VICTOR HUGO
French writer (1802–1885)

CHAPTER 10

Perfume Environment Pollution

NOW WE APPROACH the core of the problem.

After all the facts are on the table, after we know that we are being manipulated against our will, the crucial question is this. What can we actively do? What can be done that will throw a spanner in the works of the health-damaging perfume industry?

The first action, of course, is to remove perfumes and all the products that contain perfume poisons from one's immediate environment. Each of us has more power than is generally accepted. We can also talk, debate, and discuss. We can register protests. We must not be led to the slaughterhouse like sheep.

In any case, from now on, with the data we have, we will be able to study the small print in detail and re-orient ourselves completely regarding the purchase of detergents, cosmetics, cleaning products and so on.

In the meantime, we have looked at many of the tricks of the perfume industry. It will, of course, do everything it can to minimize the problem so that its splendid business is not torpedoed. No company in the world will voluntarily waive billions of dollars or euros. However, at least we can ensure that poisons are no longer allowed to be sprayed in our immediate environment or our home and workplace.

You can always do something about it.

We could do the worst thing the perfume industry can imagine. We could just stop buying their products!

That would be a big blow because any advertising that the perfume industry puts out is paid for by the consumer's money added to the price of the product whenever you buy perfumed detergents, personal care products and so on.

Each of us, therefore, possesses a lot of power. The new equation is: less money in the pot of the perfume giants = less advertising and less "brainwashing" in the direction of chemistry and perfume = even fewer sales = falling sales in the long term.

If you're looking for a helping hand, you should first look at the end of your arm.

This is a beautiful proverb, which contains more than a little wisdom.

It would be wrong to wait for others to do something. Like politicians, we could wait – until Christmas, or until the cows come home, which is to say, forever. This world will only change for the better if we **do** something.

If we do not roll up our sleeves and do something, nothing happens. In the next chapter, I shall present a detailed check-list describing the ideal order of how to proceed.

Very Good News: Perfume Successfully Banned

We now know that we cannot escape perfumes and their toxins, even if we ban all the perfumes from our environment.

If we do not decide to live a hermit's life in the Himalayas, we are hopelessly exposed to perfumes. Even there, poisons would probably reach us through the rain and the wind. It is remarkable, therefore, that a few courageous activists have long ago launched citizens' initiatives in which they are vehemently opposed to poisoning by perfumes.

This is inspiring. There are already entire cities in Canada in which artificial odors in public places can no longer be sprayed and used. In Halifax, for example, the city leaders themselves have established appropriate guidelines. Halifax is the capital of Nova Scotia and home to approximately 390,000 people. It is located directly on the Atlantic Ocean, at the easternmost tip of Canada. Citizens there have started to protest against perfume. Their excellent and combative slogan reads:

"No scents make good sense!"

In public, cosmetic odors are discredited in Halifax and eschewed. In offices and libraries, hospitals and classrooms, courtrooms and buses, perfumes are forbidden. One can only applaud.

But how did this coup succeed? The background to this is that hundreds of fragrance-sensitive citizens suffered personally from all these odors. They joined together and protested. They would not participate in events that reeked of perfume. The authorities reviewed the reasons and concluded that the protestors were right. They found that evidence existed that could not be swept under the rug.

Let us head directly from Halifax to California, which has always set the pace for new movements. Here, too, people have been protesting perfumes, in the city of Santa Cruz, a town situated in the middle of California, directly on the Pacific Ocean.

There, too, perfume odors have been publicly banned in numerous places. They already have restaurants which have perfume-free areas where you can dine. So, you have a choice. You can take your meals in the normal way, wearing any perfume poisons you like, or, if you prefer, you can stay healthy in the fragrance-free sections.[1]

Just as public authorities have been banishing cigarette smokers with their poisonous smoke during the last decades, so health-damaging perfumes are already being pushed back in a few cities around the world. Citizens of Santa Cruz have initiated extensive campaigns against *passive scents*.

Santa Cruz is firmly against the passive inhalation of perfume poisons.

They point out that you are always exposed to the perfumes of others, whether you want to breathe them or not. No one can escape perfumes, because man must breathe. Just as there is the passive smoker, there is the passive sniffer – because perfumes travel through the air and are present everywhere.

How about imitating tobacco legislation, where one law was passed after another? Today you cannot smoke in airplanes and most other public places because you will damage non-smokers and subject them to becoming unwilling passive smokers. Today, it is self-evident that there are many smoke-free zones, smoke-free buildings, and smoke-free restaurants. If we all work together in the same way, one day there will also be perfume-free zones, perhaps even chemical-free zones.

The concept is exciting. Bit by bit, we could make perfume poisons vanish this way. Hopefully, perfumed air will also become a source of anger and drive the general will of the people in the right direction. We have no other choice if we are concerned about our health and the health of our children. The health of all people on Earth has been affected.

Let us cite another motivational example. Americans, who have always been freer and more liberty-minded than many other races, protested perfumes in Detroit, a city in the United States located directly on the Canadian border. Here, the authorities have already set up a perfume-free zone. The trigger was an urban clerk who felt intruded upon by a colleague's perfume. The case came before the courts, and it was decided in his favor. The consequence? All the Public Service areas of the city of Detroit are now to be declared a fragrance-free zone.[2]

Large-scale posters have already been put up in public buildings in Detroit urging municipal employees to dispense with perfumes, aftershaves, deodorants, and scented facial and body lotions. They are even against perfumed clothing, fragrant candles, and room fragrances.

Americans are not squeamish over seeking legal redress. Unlike in Germany, complaints are made at an astonishing rate. Instituting a $100,000 lawsuit, the affected parties started the ball rolling. Now, just for a moment, imagine that this example spreads around the globe.

Happily, concerned citizens have followed suit in Germany, Austria, Tyrol, and Switzerland. When judges agree with the parties concerned, the perfume industry is always threatened with losses of billions.

The conclusion is, thus, once again:

You can always do something about it.

Not only in the United States of America is the population getting aware of the urgent need for perfume-free living. Recently, in Italy, a beach service organization published a brochure with Rules of Conduct on the beach. Visitors were not only asked to behave in an orderly and respectful manner, but women were also forbidden to apply strong fragrances.[3]

So, there is hope, after all.

In Germany, the prohibition of perfumed lamp oils has already now been demanded and even enforced in some places. Furthermore, a clear indication of the harmful substances in certain lamp oils are required to be displayed more and more clearly.[4]

The people are mobilizing. The realization that perfumes contain poisons is becoming more and more established. Everywhere, people are waking up and demanding that the health of others and oneself is considered more. Something is going on.

But what is the role of our lawmakers, who should have been active long ago?

Politics is the art of doing as little as possible for the many and as much as possible for a few.

KARLHEINZ DESCHNER
German writer (1924–2014)

A Look Behind the Scenes: From Spineless Lawmakers to Efficient, Solution-Orientated Action

THERE IS A so-called EU chemicals law, but the perfume industry just laughs at it. The reason is that there are too many loopholes in it, allowing them to spray poisonous air in all directions.

In my opinion, it is undoubtedly true that, in some circles, knowledge is growing of the danger associated with perfumes. The worldwide organization Greenpeace published the facts about perfumes in various brochures as early as 2005. They even warned of the cancer risk.

Germany

The Ministry of the Environment in April 2006 warned against perfumes. They published a paper entitled, roughly: "Perfumes: When Pleasant Becomes Problematic."[1]

But what has happened since then?

Well, one could sarcastically note that, when the German Federal Minister of Health visited the hinterland of Brandenburg to count the agricultural holdings there, the Ministry also calculated how much more tax revenue would be needed to cover rising pharmaceutical costs.

But when it came to the business of warding off dangers like airborne toxins to which nowadays every citizen is exposed, nearly every day, right around the clock, oh no, let's not rock the boat!

Major taxpayers would suddenly not be contributing so much, because certain corporations would no longer make their billions.

Do you see where the crux of the matter lies?

If the legislator is not actively and efficiently ensuring cleanliness in your environment, you must do something yourself. Otherwise, you will continue to be subjected to toxins every day.

I will tell you what the legislator does wrong at the end of this chapter, as well as what is necessary to protect ourselves, our babies, our family, our fellow human beings and the environment.

Ray of Hope: USA?

In the United States of America, the first tentative steps in the right direction have begun, especially in the legal sense. Influential Congress members who are responsible for the drafting of laws were already discussing the dangers of perfumes in the year 2010.

Deputy Representative Jan Schakowsky from the state of Illinois, for example, clearly took notice of the problem when she said:

> *"There is no sensible reason why we should be exposed to potentially hazardous chemicals because they are contained in perfume, eau-de-Cologne, or body deodorants. The chemicals found in popular perfumes, the marketing of which are supported by celebrities, can have several side effects. Americans are exposed to them without knowing it. I think this is a clear demonstration of how pathetic our laws are for cosmetics ..."[2]*

In short, Schakowsky demanded that perfumes should be checked for harmful substances. Ed Markey, from Massachusetts, agreed. He summed up with this statement:

> *"A rose, by whatever name, may smell sweet, but in some cases, a sweet-smelling perfume can be dangerous. I am delighted to have teamed up with colleagues*

to introduce new legislation that makes it necessary to name the ingredients used in the perfume, which ensures that toxic chemicals are not used in cosmetics and fragrances. Consumers have a right to know what exactly is contained in the products they spray or rub on their bodies every day."[3]

In 2010, then-President of the USA Barack Obama launched a Cancer Panel. The toxic chemicals in perfumes were tracked here, too. The findings of the report were devastating to the perfume industry.

Some politicians subsequently sounded alarms and indicated possible hormone damage and cancer. Is this increased awareness at least a hopeful sign?

Well, maybe. But there are currently loopholes in the US federal legislation too. The politicians who were issuing the warnings did not act consistently enough. Or were they stopped? By whom? Was the perfume-lobby more powerful than the good intentions of those politicians? To approach this question closely would be worth a book of its own. At present, we can only conclude that, although the dangers are known, the perfume industry is still able to sell its products unhindered.

Loopholes still allow the perfume industry to refer to "trade secrets" when it comes to specific fragrances, so they do not always have to put their cards on the table, even though numerous health damages have been established without ifs or buts.

Everything still hangs in the balance. Critics who distrust these delays suspect that there was an unholy alliance between former president Obama and the pharmaceutical industry.[4] Donald Trump, the new president, has not yet commented on the problem.

Let's watch closely how this will develop. After all, the US citizens who have dared to attack the perfume industry now provide a glimmer of hope for us all.

Legislation in the Eurozone

Let's go back across the pond and take the whole Eurozone into our sights. Although there is already an EU chemicals law, it, too, is as full of holes as Swiss cheese.

A few courageous writers (Karen Duve for example), various prominent personalities (like Peter Lohmeyer) and Greenpeace (Brigitte Behrens, to name a prominent activist) have been publicly aware of the dangers of perfume poisons and have demanded a much tougher chemicals law. Not much has happened.

Even in the context of the EU, one can refer to numerous independent tests, the results of which cannot be swept away.

Blood samples from a representative number of test persons were examined by an independent laboratory in the Netherlands for the EU. The scientists screened for fifty-five highly toxic chemicals in perfumes.

The result? Sixteen of these fifty-five highly hazardous chemicals were found in the blood of the test persons.[5] It was a catastrophic result and a blow to the gut for the chemical and perfume industries.

In the meantime, a new law called REACH is being worked on within the framework of the EU (REACH = Registration, Evaluation, and Authorization of CHemicals). But alas! Already, powerful opponents are stirring. Even during its preparation period, the probable future of REACH legislation was weakened. The existence of hazardous chemicals is undoubtedly established. Although they have been found in blood and tissue, even in pregnant women, in mothers' milk and the umbilical cord, nothing has happened.

It seems that lobbyists behind the scenes once again work hard and systematically to bring down new laws in advance!

Back to Germany

Let us turn our eyes to Germany, the nation I can most nearly observe. How does it look there?

Lo and behold, the Ministry of the Environment has made some clear statements.

This office is, after all, the highest authority in terms of the poisoning of our environment. According to their statement, they are also responsible for the health of the population and have already explicitly warned against the use of air fresheners of various types in offices, shops, department stores, and medical practices.

The Agency noted in 2006 that "fragrances and aromas could be a possible cause of allergies and other intolerances."[6] Bravo!

The Agency also pointed out that certain toxins must be declared if they exceed a certain concentration in cosmetic products, by EU Cosmetics Directive No 86/768/EEC.

But we have known for a long time that the *interplay* of many poisonous chemicals, even when present only in minute quantities, can still cause new health problems. Chemicals such as limonene react with one another and produce new toxins (more on this in the next chapter).

Finally, the existence of MCS (Multiple Chemical Sensitivity) is now officially recognized. The German Ministry of the Environment admitted in the paper mentioned above, "Perfumes: When Pleasant Becomes Problematic," that existing toxicity tests are insufficient, especially since so much data is in part inaccessible. The perfume industry is very fond of talking about "trade secrets," as I have already pointed out, and very adept at it.

The German Ministry of the Environment has complained that thousands of fragrances which are already on the market have never been toxicologically examined. Only a few, incomplete tests exist for a few substances. Some experts are finally talking about a scandal.

The industry is only obliged to declare the chemical ingredients of a fragrance if purchased in vast quantities (more than 1,000 tons per year). This brings about the situation whereby many products contain undeclared ingredients and therefore escape testing.

Chemically, it is relatively easy to check for amounts of ingredient X *if one already knows* X is in the tested substance. However, if one does not know what is in it, it is incredibly time-consuming and costly. It is sometimes impossible to determine amongst the possible thousands of chemicals which are the dangerous ones.[7]

Therefore, according to the Environmental Bureau, there is a massive backlog for testing these substances.

No one except the manufacturers knows what is in some products. The Environment Agency has also drawn attention to the fact that many fragrance-containing products imported from countries outside the EU are subject only to the provisions and laws of the country of origin.

This makes the situation and the assessment of it more difficult still – indeed, it makes an objective assessment impossible in many cases. The import of products from developing countries is growing steadily. Thousands of the examinations necessary to rule out health risks are, therefore, condemned to failure by inadequate oversight by the authorities in the exporting nations.

Some officials are seemingly apathetic as a façade to hide their awareness of what is going on.

The real sufferer is the consumer. No one ever clearly told him or her that chemically produced perfumes are harmful to health. Even a doctor will rarely tell his patient this because he has been indoctrinated during his training that every illness is caused by pathogens, which must be combated with pills – allow me once again my quiet irony.

Therefore, in the case of an acute disease caused by chemically produced perfumes, he will prescribe medicines. But they do nothing to counteract the real cause. On the contrary, drugs create a lot of side effects that can make the condition even worse.

Back from the hospital bed to the chambers of our officials from the Ministry of Health and the Environment, who are genuinely intent on doing something good for the population.

Many of them initially chose this career path with great enthusiasm, sadly to discover that they often fall at many of the hurdles in their path. There are too many legal subtleties. The law is tricky.

Products that are exclusively used for spreading perfumes in rooms are classified by law as "consumer goods." To these, many legal provisions apply – for example, food regulations and the hazardous substances law.

But perfumed body-care products used by humans are considered separately as "cosmetic products" and are therefore not subject to the legal provisions concerning hazardous substances.

So, you can see the problems that arise in the legal arena!

The Scandal About "Existing Chemicals"

While authorities are promising to look more closely at new products – read "poison products" – and their producers in the future, it is all too easy to forget that by 18 September 1981 there were already around 30,000 substances passed into law as "acceptable."

The technical term for this is *"existing chemicals."*

One can hear this and be amazed. Only 117 of the approximately 30,000 existing substances were ever detailed for each material dossier (hazard sheet). Only 117 were ever examined! (Source: Ministry of the Environment) Once again: 117 out of 30,000! That's not even 1%!

In other words, we were flooded with chemicals left, right, and center, without knowing what these tens of thousands of chemical substances could do to us, alone or in combination. The chemical industry (companies who make money by manufacturing chemicals) was and still is earning billions. Government officials conveniently "forgot" to apply legislation to serve the people.

The excuses were numerous: the costs of investigation would be astronomical, nobody could afford to pay for them, etc., etc.

As a result, the politicians quickly tried to push the industry towards self-regulation. As I have already pointed out, the chemical industry, in appointing its judge, will surely not condemn itself. Furthermore, the industry, with all its professors, doctors and "experts," will invariably, in the case of legal action, start new tests in its favor.

Air pollution is not a single commercial issue but a public health issue, which must be tackled widely. There are issues of similar magnitude that had been addressed before, like smoking and automobile emissions. The German Ministry of the Environment was courageous, in the case of harmful automobile emissions, to state clearly:

"To date, the industry markets ten thousand (motor vehicle) exhausts without having tested them systematically for environmental and health hazards."[8]

So, what about tackling perfumes? Even if the tests for new substances are going to be more severe in the future and also if new legislation (REACH) is to be instituted, we still must deal with these tens of thousands of old substances that have never been investigated.

The situation could not be more clearly defined.

REACH

A few new regulations (such as REACH), seen by many as a light at the end of the tunnel, will not change much. Let us have no illusions. There will also be backdoors to escape from REACH. If a fragrance is only purchased in "small" quantities (less than ten tons per year), it can slip through the broad-meshed law nets yet again.

The Ministry of the Environment, which is an excellent institution with honorable employees, made recommendations in its internal document. These recommendations were made not very courageously, even somewhat resignedly, in their attempts to reduce room perfuming by, so far as possible, avoiding the use of fragrances to cover unpleasant odors. They recommended informing consumers in more detail about the ingredients. The trouble is that these are non-binding recommendations, you see —

they are suggestions, not obligations. This does not solve the problem. When viewed in this light, these recommendations are nothing more than trivial formulations which hardly have severe consequences for the perfume industry.

And so:

Conclusion and Proposal for an Effective Law

Existing laws and even planned changes to European legislation will not protect consumers from perfumes. So, what should happen? Well, the following would be effective:

Part 1: A bill must be passed to protect all consumers from the dangers of improperly defined chemicals in perfumes.

Part 2: Part 1 could take a long time. Until then, you should take precautions yourself (using the hints and tips you will find in the following two chapters).

The problem is a situation in which we see the assigning of a wrong *cause* and *effect*.

The "cause" position in any situation is the place, item, or person that is causing things to happen – the one calling the shots. The "effect position" is the place, object or person which receives what has been created (caused) by somebody else. An "effect" is the result of a cause, so the "effect position" is the one that follows, obeys, or is affected.

Example: An order is given. The one who gives the order is at the cause-point. The one who receives it is at the effect point.

There are of course places in between or at balance, i.e., in some situations, you are 50% cause and 50% effect, like when you hold a position in middle management where you receive orders but also give orders. Likewise, a worker at a machine: he causes his machine to perform actions, but when it comes to what has to be produced, he is the effect of the orders which come from management.

At the moment, the chemical industry, including the perfume industry, is in the *cause position*. Every year they *cause* hundreds of new products to be released on the market.

The legislature, in its *effect position, cannot* or for some unknown reason *does not* enforce its legislation and demand necessary tests. The situation must make a 180° turn. The legislature has to get back into the driving seat, i.e., the *cause position* and assume this role. But how can this be done?

The gist of the situation is clear: with old, confusing, and complex regulations, we cannot but have chaos. So, the question is: How can you build a modern, high-rise building on top of a three-hundred-year-old wooden hut which the law says cannot be demolished?

Well, in principle, the solution is simple:

First of all: Stop thinking that nothing can be done about it!

Then: Dispose of any old laws still in use!

This finally opens the door for completely new, simple, easy-to-understand and easily controllable legislation, laid down along the following lines:

The chemical and perfume industries should be obliged to provide clear evidence that a particular chemical has no harmful effects on humans, animals, or the environment. This must apply to any chemical produced, irrespective of the quantity which they sell to the market or which they wish to market in the future.

Since chemicals can also affect our genetic makeup and fertility, one point of this would have to read somewhat as follows:

Test animals (mice and rats) must not show any adverse effects on the blood count, genotype, and fertility after ten generations.

Any chemicals which have not been already investigated and which are not certified by the Ministry of the Environment as well as by the Health Office would be classified as "harmful products" and prohibited. Infringements would be punished with monetary penalties equal to one hundred times the sales generated.

More laws are not necessary. However, a clear and unambiguous **implementation regulation** would be required, which should include at least the following points:

- **Firstly**, the perfume and chemical industries would have to finance the tests and investigations necessary for this verification. The tests would have to be carried out by independent institutes under State supervision.
- **Secondly**, products from countries, which would be opposed to these provisions and which violate them may not be distributed in the EU area.

The chemical and perfume industries have danced around existing legislation to the detriment of the health of the entire population. This fact has already cost billions, as far as health insurance alone is concerned.

The costs that the population has paid have collectively amounted to thousands of years of ill-health. So, we are not talking about just a misdemeanor in the case of perfume poisons. It is a dereliction of massive proportions – one of the most incredible in the history of mankind, in fact, when one looks at it without blinkers.

Any gradual, transitional arrangement or grace period for this new regulation would, therefore, be out of place. It is not deserved.

- Therefore, **thirdly**, all existing perfumed products which had not been put on trial and tested would be removed immediately from the market.

Since such a resounding law would hardly be able to sneak in through the back door, its contents would become known long before it was passed. This would allow manufacturers of body-care and household products to change their production from perfumed to perfume-*free*.

Barriers

Now, I like to be optimistic, but I must also be allowed to be a realist and to add this: If we sit back and wait for such a bill to pass, in Brussels, London, Washington, Moscow and Beijing, simply as a result of the publication of this book, we will wait until Judgment Day.

Bureaucrats and politicians will not solve the problem so quickly. They will not take responsibility for the perfume industry today, nor tomorrow.

Let us understand this clearly. *Nothing* will change in politics unless we roll up our sleeves and do something ourselves. To hope for politicians and bureaucrats to act is about as wise as continuing to believe in Santa Claus. It is when more and more individuals rebel, when damage claims pour down on the chemical and perfume industry and when those responsible are brought to court, that something will change.

It is vital in any case to inform the relevant authorities and politely step on the toes, if you will allow the expression, of the officials. Bear in mind that most parliaments and jurisdictions around the world are now dealing with massive, cumbersome structures that are about as mobile as an Egyptian Pyramid.

We are sold down the river and betrayed if, in our naiveté, we think that anything is going to move quickly within the framework of legislation and by fighting our way through this jungle of administration and bureaucracy!

Only when individuals *do* something, only if *you* DO something, will we be able to undermine this constant poisoning by fragrance.

To which direction should we move?

If we can dream it – we can do it.

WALT DISNEY
(1901 – 1966)

CHAPTER 12

What Can You Do?

LET'S FOLLOW WALT Disney's footsteps and be inspired by him.

Imagine that you breathe fresh, clean, clear air whenever and wherever you are, wherever you walk, jog, run, stand, kneel, sit or lie, whether at home or in the office, on the way to work or in a resort, visiting relatives or acquaintances, or in a restaurant, a train station or train, in an airport building, or in an airplane, hotel or swimming pool.

Imagine the air being as clean and refreshing as above a waterfall in the mountains or as upon a hill in a forest or as over the roaring waves on a pristine surf.

It is not difficult to dream this, is it? But if we can dream it, we can also do it.

Allow me to give you some advice. If one has decided to initiate meaningful changes, one should always begin with oneself before going further. Then, perhaps, you could take responsibility for the family, followed by a group (friends and employees at work and so on) and perhaps a whole country or even the planet Earth! Doing something on an acceptable scale of increasing activity is far more likely to succeed than trying to conquer the world overnight.

It is wise to look at yourself and start with your person and your home eco-system, so to say. So:

STEP 1
Your Body
Your Health

First, "turn your broom to your rooms," as an old German proverb beautifully expresses, before you try to convert others. Here is some more information:

Deodorants:

The first thing you should do is dispense with under-the-armpit deodorant sprays. To repeat the reason – toxins reach the entire body through the lymphatic system.

Do not listen to talk about sweating and perspiration. It is often manipulative. Keep in mind that sweating is normal. It is a *health-promoting* action of the body. When we sweat, due to heat, stress, or sports, the sweat is cleansing the body. Klaus Fritz, of the *Federal Association of German Dermatologists*,[1] as well as many other experts, has noted this.

Incidentally, fresh sweat does not smell bad. It is the later decomposition by bacteria that produces an unpleasant body odor. Anyone who suffers from perspiration should adopt a more intensive body hygiene regimen and shower more often. He or she should wear air-permeable clothing, preferably made from natural fibers, typically linen or silk, and should refrain from using synthetic materials. It also helps to avoid coffee, alcohol, hot spices, and over-sumptuous, rich food, as all are typically promoters of unpleasant sweatiness.

Lipsticks:

Let's take a look at this product.

Lips have only a thin epidermal layer, which is why the lips are red because the color of blood vessels are visible under this thin layer. To make them even redder, brighter and more conspicuous – red and black are sexual colors – many women (and some men) like to color their lips with lipsticks.

Unfortunately, at the time of this writing, about 98% of lipsticks are perfumed! Most likely, the one color you would like is not available at all in a perfume-free edition.

Lipstick-perfume poisons the wearers by permeating the thin skin of the lips.

Additionally, lipsticks contain other ingredients that are not healthy. Brands containing paraffin/petroleum products and silicones should be avoided. Paraffin can deposit itself in the liver and lymph nodes, even in a mother's milk.

The logical answer? Do without lipstick!

Dr. Esser, a Natural Hygiene doctor from Palm Springs, Florida, my good old, late friend, who taught me everything about fasting, suggested natural oils instead of lipsticks. You can choose olive oil, or whatever your favorite might be.

If colored lips are still hip (as in specific acting roles), it is recommended that you switch to natural cosmetics.

However, there is a small catch. Some manufacturers advertise their products by pointing out that they contain *natural oils*. However, they conceal the fact that paraffin wax has also been secretly used. Do you understand? Be aware! The concealment strategies regarding cosmetics knows no limits.

⊶⇒ ⇐⊷

***Only for the expert
and those who want to know exactly***

*Allergens in lipsticks are the fragrance components
citronellol, citral, eugenol, and geraniol.[2] Also, musk
compounds are to be avoided.*

⊶⇒ ⇐⊷

Anyone not well informed about lipsticks and cosmetics, therefore, is almost always led around by the nose. A whole *book* could be filled about the right lip care and many deceptive maneuvers.

You should advise people to dispense with cosmetics whenever it is possible. Perfume and cosmetics companies are now doing everything they can to confuse the consumer and entice them with words like *organic, natural, or biological*. Ha! No words are currently more abused than these!

Some substances in a product may indeed be natural, but a cloak of silence is spread over the other, toxic substances in the same product. They are not even mentioned, as already stated. So, avoid products containing paraffin, petroleum products or silicones.

⊶⊷

Only for the expert
and those who want to know exactly

Behind the words, paraffin/petroleum product/silicone, substances such as microcrystalline wax, dimethicone, petrolatum, mineral oil, ceresin, polyisobutene, and polydecene are hidden.[3] These are all poisons, which should be avoided as much as possible.

⊶⊷

Moreover, it is easy for the perfume industry and the chemist to invent and introduce new chemical compounds tomorrow and to label them with some great-sounding name with which to impress the unwary. This is nothing less than a war, an economic war to which we are exposed – and, for the "enemy," all is fair in this war.

"Natural" Products

Quote from a fine businesswoman in the jewelry industry:

> *"I write organic or natural product on it, and that makes it easier to sell."*

This is all there is to be said, as mentioned above. No other words are so deviously used as a *biological, organic,* or *natural product.*

Nowadays, it has become so widespread but known, that it has become necessary to create a new word: "washing" or "greenwashing". So, the whole thing is nothing more than a psycho-trick of the advertising psychologists to put up the image of being or operating environmentally conscious, environmentally clean, pure, natural and the like.

Soap, shampoo, or even lipstick do not grow in nature. Chemical interventions are always necessary when it comes to conjuring up a product such as soap or lipstick, allegedly from a material occurring in nature.

We should realize this: Not all of the chemistry should be demonized. It is only the irresponsible handling of toxic elements that is our concern here. The manner of processing and the number of ingredients and their properties are therefore significant. The quality of a final product can range from acceptable to very toxic, depending on how the formulation was created and how it was processed.

A 100% natural product will not be available if it has to be storable and durable. "100% natural" will only work in cosmetics if you were to peel a mango, for example, and vigorously rub the inside of the skin on your skin, which is very refreshing.

So, if you're looking for alternatives, be as suspicious as a detective. Bear in mind that most of the health-threatening fragrances cannot be identified from the list of ingredients on a product. Remember again that the EU allows the manufacturers to hide all kind of chemicals behind the terms "fragrance" and "perfume." So, you had better back away the very moment you see the words "perfume" or "fragrance" in the ingredients list.

Additionally, it would be a good habit to avoid any product which you don't need.

Essential Oils

Even essential oils can sometimes trigger allergies.

"How is that?" you may wonder incredulously. "Essential oils are a natural product, aren't they?"

OK, let us look at an example:

In the "essential oil" of most citrus fruits, we find the substance *limonene,* which has the characteristic smell that we recognize as coming from lemons and oranges. Citrus oil, especially pressed from the fruit skins, can contain 65% (in the case of lemons) and over 90% (in the case of oranges) of this natural substance, limonene.

But *limonene* can irritate the body. In other words, it can trigger allergies, as even the Wikipedia encyclopedia (and the author Karlberg, who is quoted there) reveal. Yes, essential oils can be safe because they come from nature. But the nature of their chemical components is not always stable. They react with all sorts of other elements in their environment. In the case of limonene, they can form an allergen.

Even if most of these essential oils are harmless, there is one vicious element in them: their scents are very dominant and therefore cover up any bad and dangerous odor in the room. So, you won't smell bad and dangerous ones, but you will still inhale them!

Technically, essential oils confuse the instincts that would normally warn you against danger.

Therefore, my best advice is: Regarding the occasional enjoyment of the pleasant smell of a purely natural essential oil, o.k. But beware of using such oils for long periods or in high quantities. And do not make it a permanent habit.

What your body needs is clean, clean air. Nothing else. The more you pollute the air, the higher the risk of confusion and sickness in your cells.

Cosmetics and Body Hygiene

Because of the numerous possibilities of poisoning yourself, I recommend, first of all, to say good-bye to the mania of pasting any number of different treatments and remedies on your skin every day.

We already overuse our bodies with environmental pollution from industry, vehicles, old power plants, and old heating systems, etc. ... and on top of that, we add perfume poisons, perfume poisons, 24 hours a day, around the clock perfume poisons.

What do you think weighs the most?

To answer it bluntly: No one has the right to point their finger at any other as long as one poisons oneself with perfume every day, every hour, every minute!

Johann Kellerer

Advice:

Buy PERFUME-FREE products from trusted manufacturers.

And use only a few products. Shampoo, soap, and toothpaste – I do not need more inside my own four walls. When I go on a journey, I even consider soap and toothpaste to be enough. With a good soap, I can also wash my hair from time to time. Women have higher demands, I know, especially with long hair.

As far as the world of men is concerned, I am not a friend of shaving creams and this is not just because 100% of them are perfumed! In my opinion, this is the most absurd product in the world. Every ordinary soap does the same job. It is more accessible and much more environmentally friendly. As for lipstick, perfume, toner, skin creams, lotion, and conditioners for men – do not let the advertising psychs lead you around by the nose!

Once you have eliminated all the perfumes, "stabbed them with the dagger and hacked them down with the sword," if you will allow the martial expression, and after you have moved to perfume-free products, you will have made the first step.

Your level of responsibility towards your own body will have increased considerably.

Fragrance-Free Household
(See hereto the checklist in chapter 13.)

The "Fragrance-Free Household" checklist (in the last chapter of this book) is essential. It can be extended and supplemented as you find appropriate. Successfully doing this checklist ensures that, in the future, no perfumes will enter your body – at least, not at a dangerous level. With this checklist, you also allow your body to get rid of old toxins.

In the case of acute problems, it is advisable to do a detoxification. See the checklist "Fragrance Detox Program" in the last chapter.

STEP 2
The Health of Your Family

A little wisdom: rarely, or perhaps never, does one do something good to others without also simultaneously doing something good to oneself.

The best way is to give this book to your friends and family members, work colleagues, and colleagues. In this way, genuine enlightenment will quickly spread by word of mouth. Such action also opens an inspiring perspective. If each of us becomes enriched ourselves intellectually, and then inspires *a single another person*, a domino effect immediately ensues.

Do you have a life partner? Or even children in the household? Then I suggest you have fun implementing the "Fragrance-Free Household" checklist together.

CAUTION: some people will be opposed to all of this, based on stubborn principle. Such people will fight against this planned action.

What to do in this case?

Provided you have tried to the best of your knowledge to convince your partner of the importance of these steps and provided your partner has read this book and provided your partner is against completing this checklist, then this would be the time to realize that you should have a serious conversation regarding this matter. If that turns out to be fruitless, consider whether your partner is the right one for you, sorry to say!

Ultimately, in my view, separation is better than a life with poisons, which can have considerable consequences, as you now know.

How should you behave in the case of disagreeing teenagers? Well, with my daughter, I had this problem especially since one or another product which she did not want to live without did not exist in a perfume-free form on the market.

I admit that in this case, at that time, I could not wholly avoid a small compromise here and there. Meanwhile, however, she has long since left home. Today, every time I visit, I am delighted to see how much she has ultimately listened to my advice on this subject. Now, she lives an utterly perfume-free life.

Once you have mastered this level in one way or another, you will have a home where you can breathe freely and deeply.

The presence of perfume and chemical poisons in your immediate environment is thus significantly reduced.

Owing to constant contact with perfume toxins from a third party, you had been degraded thus far to the position of a *Passive Sniffer*. Now, this should be a thing of the past.

STEP 3
Your Group

Regarding groups, I wish to direct your attention to your workplace, your sports club, and all the places where you spend time with business partners and with friends. Considering that about a third of your life is spent at a workplace, it is necessary to keep this area in good condition, to ensure that the air that you and others breathe is clean and free from perfume sources.

This step does not require a checklist. Just talk about it from time to time. If you have had great health gains, mention them to your acquaintances and work colleagues.

If you have a good relationship with your boss, talk to him or her about it. Make it clear that good, clean air will increase productivity. Conversely, if the air is polluted by perfume and similar dangerous chemicals (cheap cleaning agents), employees' performances will deteriorate. Sickness reports will accumulate.

In the following chapter, you will find a passage headed "*Alcohol, Smoke and Perfume Ban*" that should be included in every set of workplace rule. Use this as an inspiration. If you are the owner or the managing director, for example, you should include this or a similar passage in your company regulations.

But what do you do about stubborn resistance?

Remember the following sentences again:

You can always do something about it.
Something can always be done about it.

In principle, however, you will find out that 90% of all people will quickly and easily be on your side. Why? Who is not interested in doing something for their health? One must be mentally ill to a certain degree if one loves to poison oneself and others.

More data on this follow in the next step.

Let us conclude these first steps.

If you *do* all that I have recommended, then you will have already really changed something.

You are also using your mind, and so belong among those people who can *act decisively,* which is an exception today. In this case, I can only applaud you.

But in fact, you can still do a lot more. You can pursue it further, to bring these perfume poisons to an end. You can take on responsibility on a larger and larger scale.

If you decide to do so, you are among the top ten percent of the top one percent of the population. You do not close your eyes tightly or put your head in the sand. You are a rebel, in the best sense of the word. In this case, you are actively encouraging improvements to everyone. Then you fight for a whole country and maybe even for the human race.

If you belong to this category, what could you do?

STEP 4
Humanity

I am not a friend of war and strife. It is always a good idea to try good, constructive communication first, to appeal to reason, and to bring about change using amicable methods. Most people recognize very quickly that it is to the benefit of *all*.

Only when polite measures to bring about understanding don't bear fruit should you resort to other means.

Never forget: You have rights. You are not obliged to let yourself be poisoned.

Do you remember the examples from Canada and the USA? Why not go the same way? Claim your right.

In this case, you should hire an attorney. All the aces are in your hand. Find a good lawyer and a good toxicologist. Demand a right to clean air.

If a toxicologist can prove that a perfume product has caused damage to your health, you hold all the trumps. In this case, take action against the manufacturers and ask for compensation. The law is on your side. As soon as there are a few like-minded people, it is not difficult to bring citizens' initiatives and other movements to life.

Everything starts with a single person who makes a decision.

You can also address individuals, companies, or authorities directly. You can write letters, including *public messages*, which are published here and there, on the internet or in print, and which will draw attention.

Below, you will find excerpts from various texts (letters, e-mails, protest letters, but also letters of bibliographic information to like-minded people and so on) which I wrote to draw attention to perfume poisoning. Further examples will soon be available on **www.perfume.info**.

Further examples of simple actions you can do are listed at the end of the next chapter under the headline of "Your Real Power."

CHAPTER 13

Checklists and Text-Templates

IT CANNOT BE ruled out that your quality of life today is affected by perfume poisons. These are currently estimated to reach about 90% of all humanity.

If the people, organizations, and governments that you are dealing with act reasonably and for the benefit of all, you can sit back and relax. It gets unpleasant, even dangerous when you are dealing with people, organizations, or governments that do not consider their health and far less the health of others. Our quality of life is severely affected if there are organizations that bribe with billions of dollars and knowingly cause diseases.

The following checklists, programs, and suggestions are intended to allow you to turn the tables and make changes step by step, as far as poisoning by perfume is concerned.

I do know that there are many other unpleasant situations on planet Earth, ranging from drug abuse and human trafficking to warfare. Nevertheless, let's do what we can do at this moment to make a living on this planet a little less dangerous.

Checklist: FRAGRANCE-FREE HOUSEHOLD

1. Decide to forgo perfumes in the future.

2. Clear the largest table in your house or apartment.

3. Place a large trash can next to the table. If you have a magnifying glass in the house, get it, because you might have to read the small print.

4. Collect from every room in your household all the perfumes, cosmetics, soaps, and sprays, as well as anything containing cleaners and washing powders. Then, any further containers from the bathrooms, kitchen, closets, laundry room, cosmetics cabinets, dressing table, etc.

    Put them on the table.

5. Sit down and count how many objects there are on the table.

6. Firstly, pick up every container of pure perfume and throw it into the trashcan, no matter how beautiful and noble the bottle may be and how expensive it was.

7. Next, sniff the other containers without opening them. Whatever smells like fragrance ... this is garbage ... away with it into the trash!

8. It's time to go and get some fresh air (outdoors or on the balcony or at the window). Take some deep breaths to internalize the feeling of fresh air again.

9. Go back to the table. Open each of the remaining containers, one by one, and smell each. Does it smell of fragrance? If so, it's garbage ... into the trash can with it!

10. What should now be left on the table are those containers about which you are uncertain as to whether they contain fragrance or not. Read the list of ingredients and use, as necessary, your magnifying glass.

    If you discover there the word perfume or fragrance (also "parfum," "aroma," etc.) ... trash it!

11. Counting. How many containers containing a perfume ingredient are still on the table? Zero? Good! Otherwise: Repeat steps 8 and 9. If you are lucky enough to find even one product without any added perfume ... congratulations!

12. Now, arm yourself with the trash can and go to all the bathrooms.

    Collect all air fresheners, fragrance dispensers, toilet-rim blocks ... into the trash with them!

13. Check the toilet paper by smelling it! Does it smell of perfume? (Some manufacturers seem literal to want to kiss your a$$ nowadays). *Kick* their a$$ ... off with it into the trash can!

14. A shortlist of where other fragrance sources could be found:

   - Scented candles (about 98% of all candles in our shopping "paradises" today contain fragrances) ... trash!
   - Fragrances in air purgers ... trash!
   - Air "fresheners" and fragrance dispensers in the automobile ... trash!

15. Do this immediately! Empty the contents of the trash can into the garbage container outside your household. This waste is mostly hazardous waste. Please dispose according to the regulations of your country.

16. Next: Open all the windows and doors and thoroughly ventilate your home. Do this from now on regularly at least twice a day for between ten minutes and twenty-four hours, as weather and safety conditions allow. In summer, all my upper windows are usually open all twenty-four hours, the lower ones only during the day.

17. Go shopping.

    Shopping tips:

    - Go to your nearest drugstore and ask them for fragrance-free household and body care products. Go to another one if they do not have any.
    - You may have to look for organic shops. They sometimes sell both organic food and other eco-friendly products.
    - Or you may have to check on the internet to find a producer in your vicinity.
    - Stock up your home with functional, fragrance-free body-care products and household cleaners.

18. After you have done all this: pat yourself on the back! Congratulate yourself!

Checklist: FRAGRANCE DETOX PROGRAM

1. Fully and honestly complete the checklist FRAGRANCE-FREE HOUSEHOLD.

2. Set up a daily **outdoor** activity for about three to six hours per day for at least a week (the more and more prolonged the better) **in clean air**.

   Whether you walk, swim[1], jog, ski, play soccer, do gardening, cycle or sled down a slope is up to you. Whether you do this at a beach, forest, meadow or park is up to you. Just choose a venue where there are no environmental toxins, but clean, fresh air instead!

   And if you encounter any stiff old lady of rigid opinion encased in a vapor trail of indescribable perfume so strong that sharks and dolphins, wolves and deer alike flee from her headlong, feel free to tell her that it is entirely irrational and dangerous to her health to shroud herself in such a cloud of perfume and she had better *literally* taken a hike – for enjoying the "fresh" air.

   It is, of course, essential to be mindful of what you drink and eat. Nutrition is a field of data about which one could elaborate for eons. (See the text under the

---

1 If you go swimming, do not go for an indoor swimming pool, because there you are liable to pull chlorine chemicals into your lungs and that kind of toxic intake we do not need right now.

heading "Body Depressions, The Remedy" in Chapter Eight, "Perfumes, Psyche and Psychoses").

But first things first! The most important thing is to breathe good, clean air!

As already stated in the foreword, without food, you can survive, depending on how much fat reserve you have, from one to three months. This ability inherent in a body is how people can fast without ill effects for some time.

Without a drink, as in an emergency, we can go five to seven days, and then it becomes life-threatening.

Without air? A minute or two!

This should make it clear to you that breathing clean, fresh air is priority number one. Air is the most important element that your body needs to survive.

The equations are simple. The more food and drink is contaminated, the more your health will be endangered. The same is true for the quality of the air that you breathe into your body.

If, after a week, the above three steps do not bring about a significant improvement in your well-being, then follow this up with the one or more of these actions:

3. Body Detoxification

Fortunately, there are numerous methods available. There are already unique detoxification cures for single organs!

The use of a sauna is helpful. Poisons can be easily excreted through the skin. The skin is a large organ that can massively catapult toxins out of the body. They are sweated out. There is a lot of information available on how best to use a sauna.

If you are physically fit, you can sweat properly through high-intensity sport. This activity has the advantage that, as long as this sport is not exercised in a polluted venue, you will also get a lot of good oxygen into all of your body's cells. However, avoid fitness centers, where the air is usually quite polluted with perfume and cleaning chemicals.

The best, of course, is fasting. This method is extremely suppressed by the health industry (pharmaceutical companies, clinics and doctors) simply because it does not bring much money.

There are numerous variations of fasting, ranging from juice fasting to the standard fasting, which means that you only drink water and eat nothing at all. So, you only breathe air and drink water.

To fast on your own may be difficult for some people. It is better and much easier to fast in a group under medical supervision. There are health centers which specialize in fasting.

TEXT TEMPLATES

These are examples of workplace policies, protest letters, and also letters of affirmation to like-minded people, etc.

A clause in a Working Regulation:

Alcohol, Smoking and Perfume Ban

In the factory and on all construction and assembly sites, employees are prohibited from consuming alcohol during working hours. The company fundamentally rejects any indirect or direct liability for damages in connection with and as a result of alcohol consumption by employees, even in small quantities. Smoking is banned throughout the office area and project sites, except in designated areas. Any transgressor is personally liable for damages resulting from any infringement. According to recent reports from Greenpeace and the Ministry of the Environment, chemicals in fragrances have a negative impact on alertness, well-being, and health. For this reason, a ban on perfumes applies to construction sites as well as to the office.

Employees are also asked to use perfume-free hair shampoos and detergents at home since the fragrance particles contained in them will remain on hair and clothing and are therefore taken everywhere, i.e., worn in the office. Cleaning companies must work with perfume-free cleaning agents. It is forbidden to put on or hang up perfume dispensers. This also applies to all vehicles.

Email to a Business Partner Before a Meeting:
Dear …

…

May I ask you a favor? I know that chemically produced perfumes are poisonous. I am therefore an opponent of wearing perfume, and we maintain a perfume-free office. If you usually wear perfume (or Eau-de-toilette, Cologne, or the like), please could you refrain from using it for our upcoming meeting?

Best regards,

…

Letter to the Manufacturer of Perfumed Baby-Oil Wipes
Dear Sir or Madam,

You sell three different baby-oil wipes.

However, all three are perfumed.

Even though perfumes are harmful to one's health, they also smell obtrusive. We want to save our baby from being conditioned to perfume as a child. We are sure that we are not the only parents who think so.

It would be appreciated if you could keep at least one of your products perfume-free.

Best regards,

…

Johann Kellerer

Notice to Room Service in Hotels
In three languages (for holidays and business travels):

ENGLISH
to: ROOM SERVICE
from your guest: ....

I have the following request:
Please do not clean this room during my stay with anything other than a broom, vacuum cleaner, and wet cloth.

Please do not use any chemical cleaners here.

Why? Nowadays, almost all soaps, shampoos, washing powder, cleaning liquids, etc. contain perfumes.

I am strictly against perfume/fragrance/chemical scents.

Why? Because many particles in perfume are highly poisonous.

That surprises you, doesn't it? Let me refer you to the following websites, where you can find scientific data about the toxic danger of perfume:

www.perfume.info www.greenpeace.com (search for "perfume") www.umweltbundesamt.de (change to English and then search for "perfume")

The most important thing for health and wellness is a good, clean, fresh air. So, please, keep perfume out of this room during my stay.

Thank you very much!

DEUTSCH (German)

an: ZIMMERSERVICE
von Ihrem Gast: ....

Ich habe die folgende Bitte an Sie:
Bitte reinigen Sie während meines Aufenthaltes hier dieses Zimmer nicht mit chemischen Reinigern/Flüssigkeiten und dergleichen! Machen Sie Ihren Job allerhöchstens mit Besen, Staubsauger und einem nassen Lappen!

Warum?
Heutzutage enthalten nahezu alle Reinigungsmittel, Waschpulver, Seifen, etc. Parfümstoffe.

Ich bin strikt gegen Parfüm und chemische Duftstoffe.

Warum?
Weil viele Partikel in Parfümen höchst giftig sind!

Das überrascht, nicht wahr? Wissenschaftliche Daten zu der gesundheitlichen Gefährdung durch Parfum können Sie im Internet nachlesen unter:

www.perfume.info
www.greenpeace.com (im Suchfeld "perfume" eingeben)
www.umweltbundesamt.de (im Suchfeld "Parfum" eingeben)

Das wichtigste Element zur Gesundheit und zum Wohlbefinden ist gute, saubere, frische Luft.

Bitte bringen Sie deshalb während meines Aufenthaltes keine Parfümstoffe in dieses Zimmer.

Herzlichen Dank!

Johann Kellerer

中文 (Chinese)

致: 客?服务

来自您的住客: ……………………………………………

我有个请求:

在我居住期间, 请不要使用任何带化学性质的清洁用品/清洁液来打扫这间房间. 最好只使用扫帚, 吸尘器和湿抹布来提供您的服务.

原因?

现在几乎所有的肥皂,洗发液 洗衣粉, 清洁剂等清洁用品都含有芳香剂.

我坚决反对使用芳香剂/ 香水/化学香料.

为什么?

因为在芳香剂中的成分大多具有非常大的毒性.

这可能会让您很惊讶,是不是? 您可以用以下网址查询

在这些网页里您可以阅读到很多由于芳香剂而导致的健康危害的科学数据.

www.perfume.info

www.greenpeace.com 在这里搜寻 "perfume".(英文)

www.umweltbundesamt.de 在这里搜寻 "Parfum".(德文)

对健康和舒适最好的重要因素是干净,新鲜的空气.请在我居住期间不要让芳香物质进入这件房间.

非常感谢!

Letter to a Manufacturer Who Promoted "Organic Shampoos":

Dear Sir or Madam,

With this letter, I am returning three shampoos with a request for the amount of .... to be refunded to the account specified below. The reason is that each of these shampoos contains chemically manufactured perfumes. I consider it appalling that you sell such poisons under the guise of the word "organic."

According to your appraisal and descriptions, I had expected to receive perfume-free products or products containing only organically grown ingredients.

As of now, I prefer to buy from another manufacturer. However, I will gladly order from you again as soon as you offer real, perfume-free soaps and shampoos.

Best regards,

...

Johann Kellerer

Letter to the German Foundation WARENTEST (Product Test):

Ladies and Gentlemen!

Recently, I ordered two ionizers (air purgers) online from the company ... and received them promptly. I wanted to use these devices to improve the air in the rooms of my two children.

The moment I opened the box, a strong smell hit me. It stank of the cheapest "petroleum plastics" – or by whatever this penetrating smell is caused.

The second unit was the same. The products are called [...] and have the product identification numbers [...]

Whoever buys these products and places them in their children's rooms will only achieve the opposite effect of air purification – heavily contaminated air which we will all breathe, instead of the desired result (better air for breathing). Toxic chemicals, presumably plasticizers, are the reason for this. On a label, the country of origin was identified with "Made in China." I hope you can act upon this to prevent the distribution and import of these harmful products.

Best regards,

...

(On the same day, I returned both ionizers to the seller. I hope that their quality control department has by now put a stop to such products and is now importing only non-emitting, non-criminal products.)

Please never let us forget to validate those who are manufacturing eco-friendly, valuable products:

Letter to a Perfume-free Manufacturer:

Dear Sir or Madam,

Thank you very much for the fact that you have launched the "Sensitive – without Perfume" detergent.

I can only applaud your initiative. In our household, our laundry now feels quite different, because perfumes contain poisons.

Once again: thanks. Keep it up!

Kind regards,

…

Your Real Power

We could go on and on. Please recognize that by these seemingly mild letters, one can certainly bring about some reaction. Few people realize how much potential power they possess. We can all communicate, open our mouths, talk, write, and draw attention to our point of view. Each of us can exert a tremendous influence – provided he or she communicates. This influence is much higher than we sometimes realize.

There are numerous ways to intervene and to take up the cause for a clean environment. Decide on an activity that appeals to you and which gives you pleasure.

Getting an active citizens' movement off the ground is perhaps not everyone's cup of tea. But each one of us can protest. We can express ourselves. We can communicate our opinion and thus make a difference.

Some simple examples of this would be:

Write a positive review of this book on the internet.

Recommend this book to relatives and friends.

Donate to perfume.info, the nonprofit organization that owns the rights to this book. All profit from the sales of this book and donations go towards spreading the word about the dangers of perfume.

It is amazing what happens when some courageous, respectable citizens start to speak their mind.

So, this is the true message of this book: *talk* about perfume poisons. Clean it up! You have unbeatable arguments. Your communication can change the world a little bit for the better, even if you begin with a move of the smallest degree. Everything great was initially small. Like a stone that you throw into the water which creates larger and larger ripples, you can also change something, much more than you realize.

Something can always be done about it.

You can always do something about it.

A word to environmental activists and campaigners

Thank you for your valuable work. Keep pointing your finger at industries that pollute the air, water, and soil. And please also target the perfume industry in your future campaigns.

CHAPTER 14

And where is Cindy?

SORRY, I ALMOST forgot about Cindy, with whom we became acquainted in Chapter 4.

Let's look twenty years into the future; let's go on a journey with a time machine and let's meet and interview Cindy, at age fifty:

Zzzzzzzzzzt ... 2045!

"Hi, Cindy. How are you?"

"To be honest, not very well."

"Feel free to tell me, please."

"Well, I've just seen the doctor. He's diagnosed breast cancer. It seems like I'm spared nothing in life. I am twice divorced. Never found my Mr. Right. My nephew committed suicide ... I guess that was down to the side effects of the many psych drugs he had to take."

"That's terrible. Sorry to hear it".

"It's as if there's a health curse in our family. My own two babies have suffered years of eczema, asthma and now allergies. The baby of my dear cousin died of SIDS* ... and now me ... cancer. Oh, God! What have I done that you punish me so much?"

⊷⊨⊜ ⊜⊨⊶

* A note about a real serious situation:

One of the less well-explained tragedies of infant life is SIDS (Sudden Infant Death Syndrome). Until now, no clear and definite cause has been identified for this. Research is moving in many directions, but nobody has included the possibility that sensitivity to chemicals could be the killer:

- chemicals from strong and foul-smelling cleaners are applied liberally in many hospitals;
- chemicals such as those in washing powder and especially from the fabric softeners that conscientious mothers apply liberally to their household laundry.

(By the way, there is nothing at all wrong with being hygiene-conscious, provided you use perfume-free cleaning and body-care products. Just beware of cut-price "perfume-free" washing powders ... cheap products from certain countries. Otherwise, you'll have a horribly stinking, dangerous, chemical-vapor trail around your house.)

I would strongly advise any future health-service investigations into potential causes of SIDS to include some research in the following two directions:

1. Pick out by statistics the five hospitals where the most SIDS cases occur. Check the air and ventilation conditions at the times when their rate was at its highest levels. It won't be easy. Of course, you can also measure air pollutants in the hospital's air now, and you should do so. By interrogating staff, you can estimate how it was when the SIDS were at their peak.
2. Make a list of the most recent fifty cases of SIDS that occurred in private households in the country. Make inquiries accordingly and determine whether unwitting use of damaging chemicals, including perfumes, could have been a contributory factor.

With the above, I have no intention of putting the grieving parents in the spotlight of the investigators. They are victims just like their dead babies.

⊷═◎ ◎═⊷

As for us, let's quickly go back to Cindy before we lose her:

"Well, how about giving God a chance to make you happy?"

"What do you mean?"

"You just complained that God had punished you so much."

"That's how I feel."

"Tell you what, come with me. Let's time-travel back to 2020 when you were still twenty-five!"

"Now?"

"Yes, come on, hurry!"

Zzzzzzzzzzt ... 2020!

"Nice, hey? Wow. You look pretty good at twenty-five, Cindy."

"Yes, but ... it fades away so quickly."

"Well, you'll only end up going the same way at fifty if you do the same things as you did last time at twenty-five. See what I mean?"

"Yes, sure."

"So, you need to change something!"

"Yes ... but what?"

"Here. Read this book. It is all about the dangers of perfumes."

"Thanks ... I'll read it, I guess. But I don't see how that can change anything."

"You'll see. Let's talk again in twenty-five years. Bye, Cindy."

"Bye!"

Zzzzzzzzzzt ... 2045!

"Hi, Cindy. How are you?"

"Pretty good! And how are you?"

"Fine, thanks. How have your last twenty-five years been?"

"God was so gracious and generous to me! Life was so different for me after twenty-five."

"Pleased to hear it!"

"... I've just come from my check-up. I'm in good health from head to toe. I'm so thankful that you gave me that book. Ha-ha, I did realize: to give God a chance to make me happy, I first had to change my way of life myself. And in return, he gave me my big opportunity. Remember that guy from my workplace?"

"Yes, that handsome colleague from chapter 4, right?"

"Yes. Shortly after I had done all your checklists, he asked me out, and six months later we got married. Later, he told me that on our first date, he completely fell for my natural body odor. Hah!

"And hey, look at me now! Everybody says I look like I'm no more than thirty. What do you think?"

"Yes, wow, I'm impressed!"

Thanks, and that's after having two boys and a girl – who're all healthy and happy, thank goodness. So – thank you again for this perfume book."

**Something can always
be done about it.**

**You can always
do something about it.**

CHAPTER 15

(NEW)

And if you think I have exaggerated in the chapters above, read now:

OVER 50 DEATHS!

The following message just reached me via the French news agency AFP, similar text has been released by other agencies like NBC News, CNBC and others, which warrants this addendum:

"2. January 2020

The sale of numerous e-cigarettes is prohibited

The US government bans a large number of flavored e-cigarettes... The sale of cartridges with all flavors except tobacco and menthol is prohibited, as the responsible health agency FDA announced on Thursday...

E-cigarettes, in which nicotine-containing liquid is vaporized, have gained enormous popularity world-wide in recent years...

*While e-cigarettes were initially seen as a less harmful alternative to conventional cigarettes, concerns are growing among the authorities. **In the United States, over 50 deaths from e-cigarette consumption have been recorded in recent months.**"* [Boldface added by the author.]

In the subsection "The Psychologist" of Chapter 2, I pointed out a few situations in which you can, ignorantly and in good faith, stumble into the perfume trap. And if someone asked me if things could get any worse, I would have to answer today: "Yes. With e-cigarettes!"

E-cigarettes were originally not an issue in my research on perfume hazards. It was only when I recently visited someone and there were an e-cigarette and a few aroma cartridges on the table, from which I could smell the scent of perfume, that they caught my focus.

Dear smokers: No matter what advertising psychologists lead you to believe, you will get out of the frying pan into the fire when you switch from normal tobacco to e-cigarettes! Why? The flavorings in these cartridges are chemical in nature. These are perfumes. When they evaporate, they become respirable perfume particles, respirable chemicals.

I described why tobacco is less dangerous than perfume in the subchapter "A revealing comparison" in chapter 8.

Here, as an extension as to the bane of your health, a small, revealing mathematical comparison:

With a daily serving of perfume from a mixture of fragrances from shampoo, deodorant, perfumed clothing, etc., you breathe in a certain amount of perfume (chemicals).

That amount every day for 30 to 40 years ... then the chances of having cancer and dying prematurely painfully are pretty high.

With e-cigarettes, you scoop huge amounts of aroma substances (= perfumes = chemicals) into the lung system ... from there it goes into the bloodstream ... etc. ... to every single cell.

This means that e-cigarettes are more suitable for perfume suicide than the small daily dose of perfume. (May I be forgiven the sarcasm in this last line.)

CHAPTER 16

(NEW)
Corona Pandemic: What If?

ALMOST THE WHOLE world got quarantined for a virus discovered in Wuhan City, China, in late December 2019. Those that are infected and endangered totally, and the rest of all citizens partly by lockdowns.

The recommendations for this came from the international WHO (World Health Organization) from Geneva in Switzerland, the Johns Hopkins Institute from Baltimore in the USA, the NHS (National Health Service) in the UK, and the national Robert Koch Institute from Berlin in Germany. And the respective governments have passed the implementing laws.

Keywords such as coronavirus (the villain), COVID-19 (COrona VIrus Disease), lockdown (curfew), social distancing (2 meters safety distance to everyone except family members), closed schools, restaurants, cafes and the like to be remembered for a long time.

The global economy came largely to a standstill as a result, and the population, companies, and countries suffer billions of dollars in damage. Unemployment, especially in the United States, is rising steadily, and thousands of companies are at risk of bankruptcy.

Upon all of this, two things come to my mind:

a) What I experienced on a late autumn day in the 1980s, what I wrote and described over five pages a few years ago in Chapter 6 of the first edition of this book under the heading "The ignorance of Doctors about the Danger of Perfume and Respirable Volatile Chemicals."

   For a quick review and summary: It was about the young doctor who insisted that my parents' flu-like illness came from viruses that are currently "roaming the area" and did not want to take into account that it could, possibly, perhaps, by any chance, be a symptom of poisoning due to the intense color vapors present throughout the house.

b) One of the approx. 150 books on health and nutrition that I studied in the 80s: Béchamp or Pasteur, by E. Douglas Hume.

Everyone knows Louis Pasteur from pasteurized drinks (milk, fruit juices, etc.). The liquid is heated to high temperatures for a specific time to kill germs and thereby extend the shelf life. Because of these and other discoveries, the so-called germ theory is attributed to him.

Pasteur's theory (Germ Theory): Germs (bacteria, viruses, fungi, and other microorganisms) are the cause of diseases.

Almost nobody knows Antoine Béchamp. Both worked in the second half of the 19th century. They were contemporaries, even companions; temporarily, mind you. They became violent opponents because of different research results and resulting disputes, allegedly also in patent law matters.

Béchamp's theory (Terrain[1] Theory): Harmful environmental influences are the cause of diseases. And only after that and because of that do germs develop in the body.

These two theories are in stark contradiction. This becomes very obvious through the resulting and necessary research work, diagnoses, and treatment methods:

Germ Theory: You must research the entire world of germs. Then diagnose the patient to find out which germ makes him sick. And then specifically destroy this one germ without damaging the others that are still necessary for life. By which? Medications, artificial respiration, vaccinations, surgical interventions, etc. Elaborate and costly.

Terrain Theory: You find the cause in the environment and remedy it. Sounds simple and inexpensive.

---

1 Terrain in the meaning of the surrounding environment.

Since hardly anyone knows this Terrain Theory, we should take a closer but simple look at it:

The Terrain Theory

As described in Chapter 6, our body is a carbon-oxygen machine with an expiration date.

To keep this body alive, technically speaking: "To keep this machine, called a human, in operation," very specific environmental conditions are necessary. I divide them into the following four categories:

- Air
- Water
- Food
- Mentality

"Mentality" stands for and includes mental strength, courage, vitality, life energy, energetic drive, and the like.

Each group can be divided into different subcategories, but we don't want to go too deep here; we stick to the essential.

Let's look at a few examples.

Air, subcategory temperature:

The surface of the earth has a range from -71 ° C (Oimjakon, near the city of Yakutsk in Russia) to +57 ° C (Death Valley, California, US). These are the two extreme temperatures that have so far been measured on the surface of the earth, the terrain of humans.

Well, inside such a human-machine, an operating temperature of about 37 ° C is necessary. A few degrees above or below, and this machine suffers a total failure (death).

There is skin on the outside of this machine. And there are different temperatures at different points, which have a larger tolerance range than the internal temperature. The German Wikipedia says hereto: *"With pleasant ambient temperatures, the average skin temperature is around 32–34 ° C. At 15 ° C air temperature, the average skin temperature is only about 24 ° C, the finger temperature drops to about 16 ° C. The temperature in the fingers and toes can even drop to 5 ° C for a short time without permanent damage occurring."*

This means that the ambient temperatures of this machine body should not go far and not long above approx. 33 ° C or below approx. 24 ° C (if people would always walk around naked).

Any deviation from this ambient temperature range poses a danger to the functionality of a human-machine. In a nutshell: you get sick.

Air, subcategory air pressure:

The human body is adapted to the air pressure that prevails on the surface of the earth. If the air pressure is higher (far down in the sea), a body implodes. Or lower (up in space), and it explodes.

Air, subcategory composition:

A body copes well with a gas mixture that consists of about 21% oxygen and 78% nitrogen. There are also proportions of argon (approx. 0.9%), carbon dioxide (approx. 0.04%), and other gases. If the oxygen content drops below 16%, it becomes an immediate threat. If carbon dioxide rises to 10%, it becomes an immediate threat. If other elements are added, such as chemicals (like in perfumes) or carbon monoxide, parts of the machine lead to a system failure, and depending on the amount of the foreign substance, to an immediate, irreparable total failure (death).

You see, the Terrain range of the environmental conditions that can prevail is vast, but the tolerance range of the machine body is relatively small. Exceeding these tolerance limits upwards or downwards, and depending on the size of the excess, the following conditions come about:
- **Upset, Stress**
- **Feeling Unwell**
- **Illness**
- **Death**

Treatment methods based on Terrain Theory

As mentioned above: You find the cause in the terrain and remedy it.

For example, when the temperature drops below human acceptance levels – Caution: women freeze earlier than men – you just have to add warmth (warm up the room or wear warmer).

Example 2: If you spend the night in the car in the garage with the engine running (suicide intentions) (cf. page 141, chapter 6 under the heading "The Perfume Danger") and then change your mind – you just have to switch the engine off and leave the garage out into the fresh air.

Example 3: If the smog in the city scratches your throat too much – get out of the city, off to the forest for a walk. The latter does not help permanently. Only environmentally clean energy technologies can help in the long term (that, it must be said, can also be very expensive).

Example 4: Negative impact on mentality:

When you feel stressed, forced, suppressed, exploited, enslaved, and you cannot fight back - run away! Change your job position! Make new friends! Divorce! Depending on the situation. (Admittedly, it can get complicated and expensive at times.)

Example 5: 5G – I know too little about it to publish here my opinion and must, therefore, leave this to the conspiracy theorists – mostly, and hopefully, they are not right.

Example 6: If you get dizzy spells or diarrhea after every glass of water - look in the well for dirty diapers or sanitary napkins or dead toads and the like and eliminate them.

Example 7: If an entire wedding party is troubled by a headache the next day - sleep well after the hangover and do not pour Austrian wine with glycol at the upcoming wedding.

Example 8: SIDS – refer to above page 256f

Example 9: If 50% of all residents of a nursing home get a flu-like illness relatively at the same time – do an aerial examination; check for perfumes in soaps, shampoos, towels, and bed linen; check the cleaning agents for strong chemicals and the like. Eliminate the poison sources found and regularly ventilate the entire building. But at the same time, ensure pleasant air temperatures with clean, dust-free, and fragrance-free air with air humidity between 40 and 60%. And when the weather is beautiful, open all windows 24 hours a day.

Do you recognize the common denominator in these treatment methods, in contrast to the Germ Theory? Yes, exactly: Neither medication, surgery, nor vaccination is necessary.

Epidemics can be stopped exceptionally quickly. Pandemics will NEVER occur. No billion-dollar damage to the economy.

150 years on the wrong track?

There is little literature on Béchamp's work.

About 150 years ago, the entire health industry at that time sided with Pasteur. Some tongues claim that greed for money was the decisive factor: A lot of money can be made with the germ theory. With the terrain theory? Little.

When I read the book mentioned above, I thought: Interesting, it sounds easier with terrain and more logical. Why would God, or whoever invented and built bodies, make it so complicated with germs? In other words, I became more of a fan of Béchamp than of Pasteur. However, I must confess that I had one or two concerns and uncertainties regarding this issue. To fix this, I was close to studying medicine. But since this field was not among the top ten on my list of projects, I did not pursue this matter any further.

But the book, more precisely, Béchamp's theory, did not get out of my head. And now and then teachings of the same nature crossed my path:

Ayurveda, TCM (Traditional Chinese Medicine), Anthropo-sophic Medicine (founded in 1913 by Rudolf Steiner). They all operate on terrain theory, even if they do not use this word under their technical terms.

So, I left my chips in the Roulette of Health on Béchamp. Result:

I haven't had the flu in about 35 to 40 years. Also, as long as they were under my care, I never saw my children with the flu (although not vaccinated). And when I came back from a business trip with a stuffy nose and irritated air-ways, I knew that the cause was the perfume and chemicals from the hotels and the long-haul flight (10 hours crammed with 100 to 200 perfumed flight attendants and passengers and no chance a window to open) – then I had to go to the sauna and long-distance jogging through the forest a few times.

But where is the journey going with the Pasteur followers (the WHO, the Johns Hopkins Institute, the love-driven NHS of the UK, the professors at our university hospitals, 99% of our doctors, and all their patients)?

What strikes me hereto and what seems illogical to me:

We have developed technologies, you can only be amazed: manned space travel to the moon and back; unmanned to the other end of our solar system; autonomous electric cars; robotic welding systems; artificial hip joints; heart trans-plants; transform a man into a woman. All attention, and as

I mentioned in an earlier chapter: Hats off to our engineers and surgeons!

But what about our general practitioners: 150 years of Germ Theory! 150 years of research! 150 years of diagnostics! 150 years of medication! 150 years of vaccinations! **But we still have the annual flu wave???**

That is why I ask myself more than ever in the year of COVID-19: WHAT IF?

WHAT IF OUR MEDICAL SCIENCE HAS BEEN ON A WRONG TRACK FOR 150 YEARS?

WHAT IF it is so, THEN...

- the annual flu wave will keep coming back, causing many deaths and, at the same time, millions of hours lost due to incapacity to work and thus a billion dollars in damage every year.
- we are hit by economic, social, and financial disasters such as the current corona pandemic approximately every ten years.
- patients who come to a clinic for an illness will be treated incorrectly.
- hospitals, as such are a dangerous environment and cause of disease.

This is where I remember Prof. Dr. med. Franz D. Daschner:

As director of the Institute for Environmental Medicine and Hospital Hygiene at the University Hospital Freiburg, he developed unprecedented standards for a clean environment in clinics. These included cleaning methods that guaranteed fresh, clear, perfume-free, and chemical-free breathing air from the reception to the rear of the hospital. For this work, he received the »German Environmental Award« in 2000. That made him known – him and this quality standard – and that he wanted to introduce it all over Germany, but that was it then. Because that is exactly what made him the target of – the devil knows who was behind those attacks – in any case, he was torn apart in person and the standards as such then so severely that this envisioned standard unfortunately did not prevail.

Despite these hostilities, he did not allow himself to be stopped. With the prize money for this recognition, he established a foundation with which he still pursues his goals, which he describes on the website below with the words "to systematically install into the medicinal terrain environmental protection standards, as it itself is one of the greatest polluters." www.viamedica-stiftung.de

On the following page you will find his opinion on perfumes:
https://www.gesundzuhause.de/gesunde-koerperpflege/umstrittene-stoffe/

Back to WHAT IF it is so, THEN...

- the real causes of diseases will still not be recognized and will continue to grow unchecked and cause worse conditions. That said, pandemics like our Corona pandemic will appear to be puny in 50 years because there will be more and more real, big pandemics coming up.
- More and more surveillance instruments will be introduced under the "justifiable health reasons"... Goodbye, civil rights and freedoms. Hello, Big Brother watching us!
- We will be receiving compulsory vaccinations, but they will not deal with the real causes (just as little as today's flu vaccination does not safely prevent you from getting the flu). With such vaccinations, billions are thrown out the window... sorry: of course, not "thrown out." Someone gets them. Whom do they flow to? Ah, yes, the poor pharmaceutical industry.

Am I now a conspiracy theorist? NO!

No, no, no! If my fear that OUR MEDICAL SCIENCE HAS BEEN ON A WRONG TRACK FOR 150 YEARS is correct, it has nothing to do with conspiracy theory from my side. But with

a) STUPIDITY of "scientists" of the Pasteurian kind and

b) the GREED of our healthcare industry.

BUT medicine is not my core competence. I hope, I REALLY DO HOPE that I am wrong, that my powers of observation are clouded because of too much fresh, perfume-free air and that the result of my last IQ test only got 143 points because of an incorrect evaluation. Because if I am not mistaken, then we have been traveling for 150 years in a train on a track that leads straight up against a reinforced concrete wall. At that time, the journey started comfortably at about 30 km/hour. Today? The train has picked up speed: 300 km/hour.

Maybe the truth is somewhere in the middle? What could such a middle look like?

Let's say: Béchamp is right. Diseases arise from poisoning from environmental influences. This creates germs in the body.

To a certain extent, the body can deal with the germs due to a robust immune system, a strong mental strength, a young age, great zest for life, and a great urge to live. Germs may support the immune system, stimulate it to new strength. And the body becomes healthy again.

However, if the immune system is weak, the person has no mental strength, is old, grumpy, and no longer has an urge to live, the germs attack the immune system, overcome it, and push the organism towards death. This is where Pasteur's big hour comes: With his medication and vaccinations and chemotherapy, he could stop the germs in such a body and possibly even exterminate them, thereby extending the life of this person. Such an effort would only be worthwhile if this person's mental strength, courage, and vitality were restored at the same time. Otherwise, after an artificial high, it will tip over again shortly afterward.

I still see a great need for research here, necessary to bring general medicine stuck in a cul-de-sac to the scientific and technological level of success of engineering and surgery.

References

Note: The original research for this book was mainly done in Germany and the EU and partly in the UK and the US. Accordingly, most of the bibliographic references refer to German sources. Titles are therefore given in German with an English translation in parentheses. Where the source text is in English, its title is given without parentheses.

Chapter 2

1. F. Fabian, *Die größten Fälschungen der Geschichte* (The Greatest Fakes in History), Munich, 2014, pp. 53ff.
2. See "Parfüm" in German Wikipedia.
3. *Ibid.*
4. H. Wollschläger, *Die bewaffneten Wallfahrten gegen Jerusalem* (The Armed Pilgrimages to Jerusalem), Zurich, undated, p. 140.
5. "Parfüm," German Wikipedia.

Chapter 3

1. See "Aroma," "Duftstoffe," etc. in German Wikipedia.
2. *Idem.*
3. See, for example, the account of increasing perfume (and chemical) sensitivity by Kate Grenville in her The Case Against Fragrance (Text Publishing Company, 2017). More information can also be found in the work of Professor Anne Steinemann:

see Steinemann A., "Health and societal effects from exposure to fragranced consumer products," Preventive Medicine Reports 5 (2016), pp. 45-47; Steinemann A., "Fragranced consumer products: exposures and effects from emissions," Air Quality, Atmosphere, & Health 9:8 (2016), pp. 861-866; Steinemann A., MacGregor I. C., Gordon S. M., Gallagher L. G., Davis A. L., Ribeiro D. S., et al., "Fragranced consumer products: chemicals emitted, ingredients unlisted," Environmental Impact Review 31 (2011), pp. 328–333.

4. See http://pressetext.ch/news/091126022/schoenheitsbewusste-taeglich-515-chemikalien

5. (http://...beautyconscious-daily-515-chemicals).

6. See, for example, Bridges B., "Fragrances and health," Environmental Health Perspectives, 107:7 (1999), A340, and "Fragrance: emerging health and environmental concerns," Flavour Fragrance Journal 17 (2002), pp. 361–371. L. Curtis has also argued in the same publication for the testing of fragrance compounds: Curtis L., "Toxicity of fragrances," Environmental Health Perspectives, 112:8 (2004), A461, and even earlier the issue was being raised in Fisher B. E., "Scents and sensitivity," Environmental Health Perspectives, 106:12 (1998), A594-9.

Chapter 4

1. Lawson R. H., "Is there an air freshener syndrome?" Bristol medico-chirurgical journal (1963), 100:373 (1985), pp. 10-13.

2. See the studies by Wallace (1991) and Cooper (1992). Also, Rastogi and his research team carried out investigations regarding deodorants, soaps, scented sprays, perfumes, and fabric softeners. One-third of the products tested contained

toxic substances. See also www.purenature.de/inhalt/geheim_
inhaltsstoff.html (August 26, 2008).

3. See German consumer health magazine *Öko-Test*, June 1999.

4. *Öko-Test*, special issue 23, 1997.

5. See, for example, Luckenbach, T., & Epel, D., "Nitromusk and polycyclic musk compounds as long-term inhibitors of cellular xenobiotic defense systems mediated by multidrug transporters," Environmental Health Perspectives 113:1 (2004), pp. 17-24; Salvito D., "Synthetic musk compounds and effects on human health?," Environmental Health Perspectives 113:12 (2005), pp. A802-3; Luckenbach, T., & Epel, D., "Synthetic Musk Compounds: Luckenbach Responds," Environmental Health Perspectives 113:12 (2005), pp. A803–A804; Taylor, K. M., Weisskopf, M., & Shine, J., "Human exposure to nitro musks and the evaluation of their potential toxicity: an overview," Environmental Health: A Global Access Science Source 13:1 (2014), p. 14.

6. *Öko-Test* of October 2007, p. 96.

7. See test results in *Öko-Test* journals, mainly from the years 1997 onward; and their internet publications under search terms such as "cosmetics," "body care," "makeup," etc.

8. See http://pressetext.ch/news/091126022/schoenheitsbewusste-taeglich-515-chemikalien

9. See http://www.purenature.de/inhalt/geheim_inhaltsstoff.html (August 26, 2008).

10. H. Eichhorn, "Schuhcreme mit Blumenduft" (Shoe Polish with Floral Fragrance), *Sächsische Zeitung* (Saxon Newspaper), August 04, 1999.

11. "Londoner U-Bahn wird parfümiert" (London Underground Being Perfumed), *Sächsische Zeitung,* April 20, 2001.

12. See German health magazine *Natürlich Leben* (Natural Living), 2006:2, p. 42.

13. "Raumsprays können schaden" (Room Sprays May Harm), *Sächsische Zeitung*, March 14, 2000.

14. P. Hildebrandt, *Gift in den eigenen vier Wänden* (Poison within One's own Four Walls), Waiblingen, undated.

15. Amar J. Mehta et al., "Haushaltssprays können kardiovaskuläre Gesundheit beeinträchtigen" (Household Sprays can Affect Cardiovascular Health), Publication of the University of Basel, April 23, 2012

16. S. K. Müller, *Geheimnis um Inhaltsstoffe in duftstoffhaltigen Produkten gelüftet* (Mystery Revealed: Ingredients in Fragrance-Containing Products), http://www.purenature.de/inhalt/geheim_inhaltsstoff.html, August 26, 2008.

17. C. Brüggen-Freve *et al.*, "Computer Bild klärt auf: So schädlich sind Kopfhörer, Kabel, Babyfon & Co." (Computer-Bild Reveals: Headphones, Cables, Baby Monitors & the Like Are So Harmful), German magazine *Computer Bild*, July 05, 2013.

18. Magisterarbeit „Die Kraft der Düfte" (Master's Thesis „The power of Smells"), University Vienna, Carla Laganda, Dec 2013.

19. Various promotional fliers of Mercedes and *Thai Airlines magazine "Sawasdee," Advertorial, Jan 2015*.

20. *Öko-Test*, June 02, 1999.

21. "Viele Kindergärten mit Schadstoffen belastet" (Many Kindergartens Contaminated with Pollutants), dpa (German Press Agency), *Sächsische Zeitung*, June 05, 2000.

22. See http://www.mcs-america.org

Chapter 5

1. A. Hurton, *Erotik des Parfüms* (Eroticism of Perfume), Frankfurt, 1991, p. 7.
2. *Ibid.*, p. 19.
3. See "Aroma," "Duftstoffe," etc. in German Wikipedia.
4. *Ibid.*
5. See http://www.br-online.de/land-und-leute/thema/schweigen_ der_maenner/gene.xml, August 31, 2003.
6. See http://www.n-tv.de/wissen/dossier/Nicht-allein-die-Nase-riecht-article923998.html, June 16, 2010.
7. See the various publications of Professor Hans Hatt.

Chapter 6

1. J. H. Tilden, *Toxemia Explained: The True Interpretation of the Cause of Disease*, Health Research, Mokelumne Hill, CA, 1981.
2. P. L. Scheinman, "Prevalence of Fragrance Allergy," *Dermatology* 205:1, 2002, pp. 98-102, referred to in H. Sarantis, O. V. Neidenko, S. Gray and S. Malkan, *Not So Sexy: The Health Risks of Secret Chemicals in Fragrance*, published by the Breast Cancer Fund, Commonweal, and Environmental Working Group, 2010; see also www.SafeCosmetics.org and www.CosmeticsDatabase.com.
3. J. Johansen, T. Menne, J. Christophersen, K. Kaaber, and N. Veien, "Changes in the Pattern of Sensitization to Common Contact Allergens in Denmark between 1985-86 and 1997-98, with a Special View to the Effect of Preventive Strategies," *British Journal of Dermatology* 142:3, 2000, p. 490; see also A. T. Karlberg, M. A. Bergstrom, A. Borje, K. Luthman, and J. L. Nilsson, "Allergic

Contact Dermatitis Formation, Structural Requirements, and Reactivity of Skin Sensitizers," *Chemical Research in Toxicology* 21, 2008, pp. 53–69; and Heather Sarantis *et al.*, *Not So Sexy: The Health Risks of Secret Chemicals in Fragrance*.

4. De Groot, 1997 and Jansson 2001, referred to in Sarantis *et al.*, *Not So Sexy: The Health Risks of Secret Chemicals in Fragrance*.

5. Buckley 2003, referred to in Sarantis et al., *Not So Sexy*.

6. Sarantis *et al.*, *Not So Sexy: The Health Risks of Secret Chemicals in Fragrance*, p. 4.

7. For a hint of the effect of perfumes upon the human brain and psychology, see Sowndhararajan, K., & Kim, S., "Influence of Fragrances on Human Psychophysiological Activity: With Special Reference to Human Electroencephalographic Response," Scientia pharmaceutica, 84:4 (2016), pp. 724-751.

8. Sarantis *et al.*, p. 8.

9. The practice of 'greenwashing' or making products seem greener than they are, is examined in De Jong, M., Harkink, K. M., & Barth, S., "Making Green Stuff? Effects of Corporate Greenwashing on Consumers," Journal of Business and Technical Communication 32:1 (2017), pp. 77-112.

10. See *Pure Nature* 59, 2007, Idar-Oberstein, p. 1.

11. See the magazine *Allergie konkret* (Allergy Concretely), 2004:3, Mönchengladbach, p. 21.

12. *Ibid.*, p. 23.

13. See "Allergies," newsletter, at http://www.daab.de/incCF/all_news.cfm?all_news_id=58.

14. W. Mauch, *Die Bombe unter den Achselhöhlen* (The Armpit Bomb), second edition, Munich, 1996, pp. 72ff.

Chapter 7
1. All examples are from the TV documentary "Chemiefalle" (Chemical Trap) aired March 11, 2007, by the German TV station Phoenix, screenplay written by C. Hanischdörfer.
2. See Sarantis *et al.*, *Not So Sexy*, p. 12.
3. *Ibid.*, p. 10.
4. *Ibid.*, p. 18.
5. K. Langbein, H.-P. Martin, and H. Weiß, *Bittere Pillen* (Bitter Pills), Cologne, 2004.
6. See, for example (among other studies), Buckley, J. P., Palmieri, R. T., Matuszewski, J. M., Herring, A. H., Baird, D. D., Hartmann, K. E. & Hoppin, J. A., "Consumer product exposures associated with urinary phthalate levels in pregnant women," Journal of Exposure Science and Environmental Epidemiology 22 (2012), pages 468–475; Just, A. C., Adibi, J. J., Rundle, A. G., Calafat, A. M., Camann, D. E., Hauser, R., Silva, M. J., Whyatt, R. M., "Urinary and air phthalate concentrations and self-reported use of personal care products among minority pregnant women in New York city," Journal of Exposure Science & Environmental Epidemiology 20:7 (2010), pp. 625-33; Nassan, F. L., Coull, B. A., Gaskins, A. J., Williams, M. A., Skakkebaek, N. E., Ford, J. B., Ye, X., Calafat, A. M., Braun, J. M. & Hauser, R. (2017), "Personal Care Product Use in Men and Urinary Concentrations of Select Phthalate Metabolites and Parabens: Results from the Environment And Reproductive Health (EARTH) Study," Environmental Health Perspectives 125:8 (2017), 087012; Parlett, L. E., Calafat, A. M., & Swan, S. H., "Women's exposure to phthalates in relation to use of personal care products," Journal of Exposure Science & Environmental Epidemiology, 23:2 (2012), pp. 197-206; Braun, J. M., Just, A. C., Williams, P. L.,

Smith, K. W., Calafat, A. M., & Hauser, R., "Personal care product use and urinary phthalate metabolite and paraben concentrations during pregnancy among women from a fertility clinic," Journal of Exposure Science & Environmental Epidemiology, 24:5 (2013), 459-66.
7. Mauch, *Die Bombe*, p. 52.
8. Tilden, *Toxemia Explained.*

Chapter 8
1. Fact Sheet titled "Making Sense of Scents", compiled by Julia Kendall, Co-Chair, Citizens for a Toxic-Free Marin, borrowing from Irene Wilkenfeld's "Fragrance Facts," and from research contributed by Karen Stevens, Carol Kuczora, Milan Param, Richard Conrad PhD, Susan Nordmark, Susan Springer, Mary Ann Handrus, Susan Molloy, and Sandy Ross PhD. with an introduction by Andrea DesJardins titled "Sweet Poison: What Your Nose can't Tell You about the Dangers of Perfume," © 1997 at http://enviroknow.tripod.com/Perfume.html, p. 1.
2. Elliott, J. F., Ramzy, A., Nilsson, U., Moffat, W., & Suzuki, K., "Severe, intractable eyelid dermatitis probably caused by exposure to hydroperoxides of linalool in a heavily fragranced shampoo," Contact Dermatitis 76(2) (2017), pp. 114-115.
3. *Ibid.*, p. 2.
4. *Ibid.*, p. 3.
5. *Ibid.*, p. 3.
6. Candida Research and Information Foundation: Perfume Survey, Homer, AK, 1989-1990.
7. Fact Sheet "Making Sense of Scents," p. 2
8. See the (German) Wikipedia under search terms such as "Zunahme von Geisteskrankheiten" (increase of mental

disorders), and any amount of other commentary such as the BBC infographics on "Mental Health: 10 charts on the scale of the problem", anxietycentre.com, "Why is Mental Illness on the Rise?" and many other sources.

Chapter 9
1. Mauch, *Die Bombe*, p. 47.
2. See B. Ehgartner, *Dirty Little Secret: Die Akte Aluminium* (Dirty Little Secret: The Aluminum File), Steyr, Austria, 2013.
3. Mauch examined more than 2,000 patients and reached that very conclusion.
4. Fact Sheet "Making Sense of Scents," p. 2
5. "Perfume: An Investigation of Chemicals in 36 Eaux de Toilette and Eaux de Parfum," published by Greenpeace International, Brussels, 2005. Numerous references from other scientists are listed in this report.
6. "Mein Sohn hat sich mit Deo-Spray zu Tode geschnüffelt" (My Son Snooped to Death with Deodorant Spray), T. Gaedt in www. Bild.de, of February 12, 2010

Chapter 10
1. Unnamed author, "There is Trouble in the Air," *The Guardian Weekend*, September 18, 2004, p. 97.
2. *Detroit News*, March 16, 2010, as well as APN News of the same date.
3. „Starkes Parfüm vom Strand verbannt" (Strong Perfume banned from Beach), C. Frentzen, dpa (German Press Agency), Leipziger Volkszeitung (Leipzig Public News) of July 25, 2005.
4. This news of January 3, 2000, on legal changes, was published in various journals and newspapers.

Chapter 11

1. *Duftstoffe: Wenn Angenehmes zur Last werden kann* (Perfume: When Pleasant Becomes Problematic), report by the Umwelt-Bundesamt (German Ministry of the Environment), April 2006.

2. Sarantis *et al.*, *Not So Sexy*; see also http://www.safecosmetics. org and http://www.purenature.de, June 28, 2010.

3. Quoted from *"Das Geheimnis von Parfüm, Studie findet (versteckte) Chemikalien"* (The Secret of Perfume, Study finds (hidden) Chemicals) at www.purenature.de/inhalt/parfum_chemie. html, p. 3., October 2010

4. Compare numerous internet articles that appear when you enter keywords around Obama related to the pharmaceutical industry: for example, Peter Baker's article "Obama Was Pushed by Drug Industry, E-Mails Suggest" in *The New York Times*, June 8, 2012.

5. *Gifte im Blut: Vier Botschafter fordern ein starkes EU-Chemikaliengesetz* (Poisons in the Blood: Four Ambassadors Demand a Strong EU-Chemical Law), http://www.greenpeace. de/themen/chemie/nachrichten/artikel/gift_im _Blut_vier botschafter..., April 15, 2011, pp. 1-3.

6. *Duftstoffe: Wenn Angenehmes zur Last werden kann* (Perfume: When Pleasant Becomes Problematic), report by the Umwelt-Bundesamt (German Ministry of the Environment), April 2006.

7. Hence the shortness of the list of irritants and allergens so far identified positively: European Union Health and Consumers Scientific Committees publication, "Perfume allergies," 2012 (http://ec.europa.eu/health/scientific_committees/opinions_layman/perfume-allergies/en/index.htm).

8. *Duftstoffe* (Umwelt-Bundesamt report), p. 10.

Chapter 12

1. See "Wie man dem Schweißgeruch zu Leibe geht" (How to Get Rid of Sweat Odor), *Süddeutsche Zeitung* (South German News), August 22, 2000; see also the brochure "Kosmetik" (Cosmetics), published by the Verbraucherinitiative (Berlin Consumer Initiative), Berlin, Elsenstraße, undated; and information sheets from the Bundesverband der Deutschen Dermatologen (Federal Association of German Dermatologists), Berlin, undated.

2. "Lippes Kummer" (Lip Problems), C. Throl, *Öko-Test*, October 2007, p. 87.

3. *Idem*, p. 61.

Index

About the Author

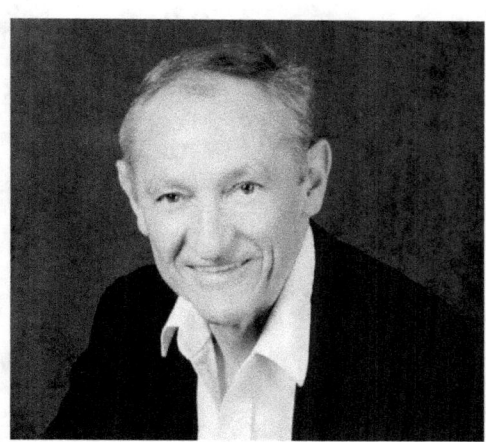

Johann Kellerer, born in 1955, graduated as a civil engineer, with a few additional semesters in philosophy and management.

In the Bundeswehr (German army) he held the rank of drill sergeant before assuming responsibility for nonprofit organizations for over fifteen years.

The 1980s saw him as an activist for organic foods and healthy lifestyles, the 90ies as developer of renewable energy projects.

Since 2003 to 2020 he has been Managing Partner of a group of companies which is active in steel and plant construction as well as in environmentally friendly energy solutions.

In 2017 he founded the UK nonprofit association perfume. info to provide information on the dangers of fragrances, operate the website **www.perfume.info** and, last but not least, translate publish, and promote this book into all the major languages of the world.